The Doctor Will See You Now

The Doctor Will See You Now

**ESSAYS on the CHANGING
PRACTICE of MEDICINE**

CORY FRANKLIN, MD

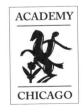

ACADEMY

CHICAGO

Published by Academy Chicago Publishers
An imprint of Chicago Review Press Incorporated
814 North Franklin Street
Chicago, Illinois 60610
ISBN 978-0-89733-929-2

A list of credits for the previously published pieces in this collection can be found
on pages 269–270.

Library of Congress Cataloging-in-Publication Data
Names: Franklin, Cory M., author.
Title: The doctor will see you now : essays on the changing practice of
    medicine / Cory Franklin.
Description: Chicago, Illinois : Academy Chicago Publishers, [2018] |
Identifiers: LCCN 2017039624 (print) | LCCN 2017043313 (ebook) | ISBN
    9780897339308 (adobe pdf) | ISBN 9780897339322 (epub) | ISBN 9780897339315
    (kindle) | ISBN 9780897339292 (trade paper)
Subjects: LCSH: Medicine—Practice—Miscellanea.
Classification: LCC R728 (ebook) | LCC R728 .F73 2018 (print) | DDC
    610.68—dc23
LC record available at https://lccn.loc.gov/2017039624

Cover design: Andrew Brozyna
Cover images: Doctor: Golden Sikorka/Shutterstock; pen: vladwel/Shutterstock.
Typesetting: Nord Compo

Printed in the United States of America
5 4 3 2 1

CONTENTS

THE PATIENT/PHYSICIAN RELATIONSHIP AND REPORTING MEDICINE

1

THE BOND BETWEEN PATIENTS AND PHYSICIANS IS IN JEOPARDY

The good physician treats the disease;
the great physician treats the patient who has the disease.

—Sir William Osler, MD

REMEMBER YOUR PERSONAL PHYSICIAN? He or she may not be yours much longer. And even if you keep your doctor, the odds are he or she is not really working for you. Soon most doctors will have abandoned their private practices and become employees of hospitals, multihospital affiliations, or the government. Only 35 percent of doctors currently describe themselves as independent, compared with 62 percent in 2008. This trend will undoubtedly continue; a medical student starting training today has virtually no chance of starting his or her own solo practice.

How did this happen, and why is it a threat to patients? The main culprits are the government and the insurance companies. As a result of the payment provisions under the Affordable Care Act (ACA), the government essentially encouraged hospitals to "own" doctors, and it is likely these provisions will remain in any modifications of the ACA. With inscrutable logic, the government pays more for the exact same medical procedure or doctor's visit if it is done in a hospital clinic rather than in an independent doctor's office. This is a strong incentive for hospitals to buy physicians and their practices. Doctors may have little alternative but to take salaried hospital positions if their practices disband. Combine this with federal rules and regulations regarding electronic records and medical partnerships that make it prohibitively expensive for all but the largest physician partnerships to compete.

Over the past several years, more than a quarter of a million doctors have been informed their Medicare and Medicaid payments would be reduced because they have not sufficiently implemented electronic medical records. Small physician practices unable to afford the capital investment are hurt the worst—just another nail in their coffin.

The government's willing partner in the dismantling of private practice is the insurance industry. Even before the Affordable Care Act, insurance companies advocated "narrow networks"—business speak for deciding which doctors patients could choose—as the means to control costs, offer reduced premiums, and broaden coverage (without mentioning the opportunity to realize higher company profits).

Put simply: one way for insurance companies to control premiums is by limiting patients' choices of doctors. These networks could change every few years; every time they do, some doctors will be shown the door. None of this bodes well for either American medicine or patients, no matter how the insurance industry and the federal bureaucracy spin it with corporate jargon like "consolidated health systems," "coordinated care delivery," or "pooled financial risk." These large consolidated health systems eliminate any possible benefit derived from local competition. Consider that when Wal-Mart comes into a community and forces out the corner mom-and-pop grocery store, the locals may be opposed, but at least everyone generally benefits from greater product selection and lower prices. In today's brave new health care world, as corporatization increases there is less selection and prices do not drop.

But there is a far more ominous implication. The centuries-old bond between patient and physician, described by Hippocrates twenty-five hundred years ago, is in jeopardy. The mutual-trust relationship is frayed when physicians become corporate (or government) employees; their loyalties are divided between their employer and their patient. How does the doctor determine how to advise or treat a patient? Is it what is in the patient's best interests, or is it adhering to performance goals and satisfaction surveys, which are increasingly being used as rewards or penalties that factor into the doctor's salary?

Fortunately, in most cases, there is no conflict, and when there is, most doctors still act in their patients' best interests. But now there is an ever-present threat the doctor will defer to a "quality improvement initiative" designed by a faceless manager in some distant corporate headquarters.

This new disconnect between patient and physician is typified by the electronic medical record. Despite never being adequately tested for actual utility, the computerized record was introduced to medicine over the last two decades at a cost of billions of dollars. In 2009 the government provided even more billions of dollars in bonuses if providers implemented the electronic medical record. The electronic record is admittedly easier to read and transmits information off-site better than paper records. But it has introduced an invisible barrier between patient and physician. Doctors now stare at a computer screen while they talk to patients and then spend an inordinate amount of time completing electronic records, time that would be better spent talking to patients. Cut-and-paste and poorly designed software templates create bad habits when doctors question and examine patients. And the records are anything but secure: millions of electronic medical records have been hacked or stolen; the information in millions more is routinely sold to third parties. Hardly a technology that engenders trust.

There has always been a love-hate relationship between doctors and society. Some physicians are lampooned as imperious jerks, and others are accused of doing too many tests and procedures. (President Obama famously made that assertion early in his presidency.) However valid these charges, one thing has always been true: with rare exception, even the most arrogant or venal physician has had the patient's best interests at heart. Can the same be said of the new business mandarins in charge of health care? With physicians becoming pawns in a much larger game, who will look out for patients? We may never again be completely sure.

2

IS IT SMART TO SKIP YOUR ANNUAL PHYSICAL?

Well, first of all, let me say that I might have made
a tactical error in not going to a physician for 20 years.
It was one of those phobias that really didn't pay off.

—WARREN ZEVON

THE POORLY TOLD TRUTH may be the most misleading falsehood. Ezekiel Emanuel, a leading American physician, provoked national debate in 2014 by suggesting that most people should not live past age seventy-five. Later he sparked further controversy, advising healthy people to forgo annual physical exams. He wrote in the *New York Times*, "Not having my annual physical is one small way I can help reduce health care costs—and save myself time, worry and a worthless exam. . . . Those who preach the gospel of the routine physical have to produce the data to show why these physician visits are beneficial. If they cannot, join me and make a new resolution: My medical routine won't include an annual exam."

The medical community has debated this issue for decades. Emanuel, displaying great assurance, relied on an analysis that pooled data from fourteen studies. He wrote, "In 2012, the Cochrane Collaboration, an international group of medical researchers who systematically review the world's biomedical research, analyzed 14 randomized controlled trials with over 182,000 people followed for a median of nine years that sought to evaluate the benefits of routine, general health checkups. . . . The unequivocal conclusion: The appointments are unlikely to be beneficial."

This is strong stuff, especially coming from an éminence grise like Dr. Emanuel when he cites the Cochrane Collaboration, a respected not-for-profit network of health experts. Unfortunately, a careful reading of the report on general health checkups reveals surprising limitations in the data of Emanuel's source—which question whether Emanuel's conclusions are applicable today. Some limitations in the Cochrane report, and the studies comprising it, include:

- Six of the fourteen studies were done in the 1960s. Nine were done more than forty years ago.
- Not a single study was initiated in the twenty-first century.
- No study included patients over age sixty-five or under eighteen.
- Five studies excluded women.

The actual median follow-up time for the patients was closer to six years rather than nine, insufficient time to prove or disprove the value of annual checkups for patients in whom chronic diseases are identified. The only studies that followed patients for more than ten years all began before 1971. Five studies did not track mortality in the patients. The nine that did all began before 1993.

An entire generation of medicine has elapsed since these studies were clinically relevant; for some studies, two generations. Is this credible evidence that routine doctor visits are worthless? Consider heart disease. Virtually all the Cochrane patients were studied when cardiac catheterization was in its infancy, when many effective blood pressure medicines had not yet been discovered, and before statin drugs became routine treatment for high cholesterol. Today asymptomatic patients found by their doctors to have hypertension or hyperlipidemia are far more likely to receive effective therapy than was possible during the study period.

For children and the elderly, excluded from this report, vaccination is more effective today than when these studies were performed. In terms of cancer treatment, most current chemotherapy had not yet been developed, and screening colonoscopy was not yet the standard for detecting colon cancer. More than half the Cochrane studies were done before CT scans, an invaluable tool in cancer management, were available. None of this demonstrates the benefit of annual doctor visits. A narrow interpretation of Emanuel's point may be valid. In healthy patients with no complaints, detailed physical examination is unlikely to detect lifesaving findings. Assuming one is healthy and asymptomatic, many doctor visits result in excessive blood testing and X-rays, merely provoking concern, leading to more testing and driving up costs.

Yet the absence of value in a comprehensive physical exam does not mean people should avoid doctor visits. Most people, even the healthy, should visit the doctor at reasonable intervals for personalized evaluation and age-specific testing and intervention. Young people should have vaccinations, developmental evaluation, and counseling. The elderly, more prone to developing chronic conditions, should be screened and also counseled about safety issues (e.g., driving difficulties, falls), memory problems, and medication evaluation. (The elderly are on more medications than ever before.)

For everyone else, routine visits to the doctor should be a serious consideration. Yearly intervals are a decent target and easy to remember. Visit frequency should be based on individual health history, family history, personal habits, occupation, and personal concerns. A complete physical exam may only be necessary if you have specific symptoms, but weight and blood pressure checks are essential, especially if you have a family history of hypertension or are African American, where hypertension occurs more commonly and at an earlier age. Cancer screenings—mammography, Pap smear, and colonoscopy—are not annual tests but should be benchmarked at regular intervals. Skin screening for cancer is important when someone has significant sun exposure, and the doctor should inquire about smoking, drinking, drug use, occupation-related conditions (e.g., repetitive stress injury), and excessive stress. All these are important to your ongoing health history.

There is no hard-and-fast rule regarding bloodwork and X-rays, other than to ask your doctor whether you need specific tests and why he or she is ordering them. The medical community continues to research appropriate indications for testing; different doctors take different approaches. Just be informed as to the whys and wherefores of the tests. Younger patients, especially, should have ongoing records of their radiation exposure history from X-rays and CT scans. We may not know for decades whether we will confront an epidemic of medically related radiation cancers.

A final word on the routine doctor visit. Just talking with your doctor, so you know he or she cares, is a good way to spend a couple of minutes once a year. Yes, time spent thumbing through outdated magazines in the waiting rooms may be tiresome (doctors have to work on that), but getting to know your physician is a good idea. It might be old-school, but trust in your doctor is a vital element of your health, and that wasn't mentioned in the studies cited by Dr. Emanuel.

3

HOW OLD IS TOO OLD?

---

*Old age has its pleasures, which, though different,
are not less than the pleasures of youth.*

—W. SOMERSET MAUGHAM

IN A CONTROVERSIAL ARTICLE in a 2014 issue of the *Atlantic*, Dr. Ezekiel Emanuel wrote, "Seventy-five. That's how long I want to live: 75 years." The controversy is not strictly because of the sentiment he expresses; many people feel the same way he does about growing old. Even Psalm 90 in the Bible describes a similar life span for man: "The days of our years are threescore years and ten [70]; and if by reason of strength they be fourscore years [80], yet is their strength labor and sorrow; for it is soon cut off, and we fly away."

Nor, to his credit, does Emanuel draw cheap attention to himself by advocating for legalizing euthanasia and physician-assisted suicide. He has always been against those movements and in favor of improving hospice and end-of-life care. But his remarks are provocative because he is one of the most influential doctors in America—a key health adviser to President

Barack Obama, as well as a brother of Chicago mayor Rahm Emanuel. When he advocates life past seventy-five is not worth living, at some point there may be public policy implications.

In the article, he wrote, "The fact is that by 75, creativity, originality, and productivity are pretty much gone for the vast, vast majority of us. . . . It is true, people can continue to be productive past 75—to write and publish, to draw, carve, and sculpt, to compose. But there is no getting around the data. By definition, few of us can be exceptions."

Before consigning everyone over seventy-five to the fate of Soylent Green (if you're under fifty, google that reference), Emanuel should be reminded what his world might look like were it not for those exceptional people over seventy-five. When he was over seventy-five, President Ronald Reagan gave his famous speech challenging Soviet leader Mikhail Gorbachev to tear down the Berlin Wall. No speech was more crucial to ending twentieth-century European Communism.

While Emanuel, a Democrat, may hold no special fondness for Reagan, in terms of political balance he need only look at Edward Kennedy, the long-time Democratic senator from Massachusetts. In 2008 when Kennedy was over seventy-five, he compared his brother, President John F. Kennedy, to Barack Obama. The senator then made the momentous decision to endorse Obama for the Democratic nomination for president at the expense of Hillary Rodham Clinton. Without the Kennedy endorsement, Obama might not have won the nomination and become president.

In his eighties, British leader Winston Churchill completed one of the twentieth century's greatest historical works, *A History of the English-Speaking Peoples*. Astronaut John Glenn, the first American to orbit the Earth, became the oldest person, at the age of seventy-seven, to fly in space. In a remarkable and underreported life, adventurer Barbara Hillary, having survived cancer, at the age of seventy-five became the first African American woman to reach the North Pole. Four years later, she made it to the South Pole, becoming the first African American woman to visit both poles.

In the *Atlantic*, Emanuel despaired of the declining contributions of elderly scientists. Yet when he was eighty-eight, Dr. Michael DeBakey, America's greatest heart surgeon, supervised Russian cardiac surgeons who performed bypass surgery on Russian president Boris Yeltsin. DeBakey practiced medicine, lectured, and wrote well into his nineties. His medical career alone spanned Emanuel's natural life span of seventy-five years. Barbara McClintock won the Nobel Prize in Physiology or Medicine when she was in her eighties for her groundbreaking work in genetics.

If any group has the right to take issue with Emanuel, it is attorneys. When he was seventy-eight, Supreme Court justice Oliver Wendell Holmes Jr. issued an opinion, familiar to every law student, that outlined the limits of free speech: he wrote that the First Amendment "would not protect a man falsely shouting fire in a theater and causing a panic." His colleague, Louis Brandeis, served on the court for twenty-three years, well into his eighties. Three of the nine current Supreme Court justices are over seventy-five. Great authors including George Bernard Shaw and Johann Wolfgang von Goethe did some of their best writing after they were seventy-five, and two of the immortal artists of the Renaissance, Michelangelo and Titian, worked prolifically until they were nearly ninety.

But put aside all the accomplishments of the extraordinary elderly. Emanuel has overstepped his bounds for reasons other than those "exceptions." Simply consider ordinary people over seventy-five—all the love and affection they give to others, as well as all the love and affection others give to them. Imagine how much poorer our country would be without that love.

Emanuel's ostensibly commonsense advice that people should not live past seventy-five brings to mind what the philosopher Bertrand Russell once wrote: "This is one of those views which are so absurd that only very learned men could possibly adopt them." Russell happened to be eighty-seven when he wrote that.

4

THE MISSING PIECES
OF BREAST CANCER

Women agonize over cancer; we take as personal
threat the lump in every friend's breast.

—MARTHA WEINMAN LEAR

MARTHA LEAR, a health care writer and advocate, has aptly charac-
terized breast cancer as a disease that not only strikes women indi-
vidually but also threatens the entire community of women. The statistics
are sobering—it is the second-most common cause of cancer in females
(next to skin cancer) and is the second leading cause of cancer deaths in
females (next to lung cancer). This year, there will be more than 250,000
new cases diagnosed and more than 40,000 deaths from breast cancer in
women in the United States.

But the news is not all bad. The vast majority of breast lumps, about 80
percent, prove not to be cancerous. For women diagnosed with breast cancer, both the number of patients cured and the long-term survival of others

have been increasing for the past two decades as a result of earlier diagnosis and more effective treatments. These figures will only continue to improve, owing to extensive research in many areas—better diagnostic modalities for early detection, improved surgical procedures, a more complete understanding of tumor cell biology and molecular genetics, and more effective pharmacotherapy tailored specifically to the individual patient. There are currently a number of promising areas, including a new understanding of the relationship between breast cancer and estrogens, a possible preventive role for vitamin D, and new drugs that might actually forestall tumors in genetically predisposed women. Compared to a generation ago, breast cancer has become a manageable and, in many cases, a curable disease.

Today much of the relevant breast cancer information is available and readily accessible, not only through your doctor's office or local medical center but also via the American Cancer Society, the National Institutes of Health, Women's Health Initiatives, and a number of valuable websites on the Internet. These are resources to take advantage of—the more you know, the less anxiety you will feel. But some observations and advice are best gleaned through the personal experiences of patients with breast cancer and the doctors caring for them.

Before writing this, I talked with two women with breast cancer who have received chemotherapy, one of whom happens to be an oncologist. I also talked to two doctors—one a local surgeon who is a national leader in the field, and the other one of the country's top breast cancer researchers. Generalizations about an area as complex as breast cancer are fraught with hazards, and some recommendations may not be right for everyone. Nevertheless, the four interviewees were fairly consistent in their thoughts. Below are some of their observations.

Be Your Own Patient Advocate

The first and most important point: If you've noticed a lump or other breast abnormality, take it seriously. Don't put off getting an answer, and don't be afraid of returning to the physician until you have an answer as to what it is. Denial remains an obstacle to early diagnosis, and early diagnosis is the key to treatment. If the lump turns out to be breast cancer, once you've been diagnosed, your life becomes an emotional roller coaster, with all the attendant highs and lows. Swings in emotion are part and parcel of breast cancer—fear of the diagnosis, anxiety waiting for lab results and tests, reluctance to bother busy physicians, and frustration with bureaucracy and insurance companies (if you're fortunate enough to have insurance). These are normal reactions, and you must work to remain in control. Coordinate your goals with your health care team. It may be an uphill fight, but it is not an insurmountable struggle.

In your initial meetings with your doctor, bring a spouse or trusted friend for support, someone who will maintain equanimity. Come prepared to assimilate lots of information by bringing in well-thought-out, written questions. Be assertive but polite regarding information you require, especially issues like therapeutic alternatives and side effects of therapy. Listen closely to what your doctor says, write down relevant answers, and don't let important details fall through the cracks. Between treatment regimens, side effects, testing schedules, and how to cope, it's easy to be overwhelmed. Ask the doctor or nurse if they can provide a written care protocol—instructions and a schedule indicating important appointment intervals, as well as dates and times of post-op care, testing, and chemotherapy. At every point of your care, always remember to speak up for yourself.

You will have no better allies than intelligent, caring physicians and nurses. Nevertheless, if your insurance and time allow, feel free to ask your physician to seek a second opinion, with the assurance it's no reflection on him or her. It's important to consider various options and opinions on the treatment of different lesions depending on your particular case. Ask whom they would go to (or send a family member to).

Breast cancer is a difficult disease to deal with and more difficult if you're alone. Make use of the best support team you have—family, friends, and neighbors. Talk to other people with breast cancer and share experiences. The Internet can be a godsend. Besides providing informational websites and support groups, it offers interactive websites where you can tell your story and learn about those of other people, from your neighborhood or other parts of the world. It's an effective way of sharing information without having to constantly retell your story. An interactive website is also a good way of keeping a diary of your experiences.

Besides complications that required hospitalization, some of the more bothersome complications mentioned by the patients I talked to were chemotherapy-induced hair loss (expensive wigs were not always better, and some support organizations offered more affordable wigs that were just as attractive, while some women simply opt for bandannas); postoperative lymphedema (arm swelling), often managed best with special massage by an experienced nurse or therapist; and skin rashes so severe they required consultation with a dermatologist.

If you have children, when they are old enough, be open about your disease. Talk to them about it and answer their questions. Once you have breast cancer, it is a part of your life forever, and it's impossible to hide from your children. Once you've told your children, discuss the situation with a responsible adult at their school.

Confidence in Caregivers

The outside world can be a threatening and unfriendly place to a breast cancer patient. The patient will interact with a multidisciplinary team consisting of physicians, surgeons, oncologists, radiologists, chemotherapy nurses, social workers, physical therapists, and others. This can be intimidating, and not every patient has a primary care doctor involved with her breast cancer care. In some centers, the primary care role has been minimized, but a good primary caregiver can be a facilitator to coordinate care. Confidence in the delivery system is crucial to the patient. (In a charity clinic where I work, some women without insurance won't go for free screening mammograms simply because they lack confidence in the centers they are sent to.) Every caregiver, especially on initial encounter with the patient, must recognize and appreciate the patient's vulnerabilities and fears and strive to win her confidence.

Both competence and a caring nature are indispensable characteristics for everyone working on a breast cancer team. Though competence is essential, most patients don't appreciate the competent but "cold" caregiver. Next to the actual care the patient receives, the most important aspect of her treatment is the information she receives and how it is imparted. Yet many studies have documented shortcomings in how professionals deliver information to patients.

Whenever possible, patients should receive bad news in person. It is generally preferable to have the patient come to the office rather than explain complicated information over the phone or via e-mail. However, the phone and e-mail have their place. When the doctor or nurse receives and returns messages from patients in a reasonable period of time, it demonstrates their concern and minimizes patient anxiety. Small gestures also can be important. Hospitalized patients appreciate the concern of a doctor who may not be active in their current care but who stops by anyway, if only for a moment to say hello.

From the time of the diagnosis through every stage of treatment, clinicians are confronted with a whole host of diagnostic and therapeutic options. Often the "right answer" is not known with certainty or is changing according to the medical literature. In individualizing therapy, physicians should explain therapeutic options to the patient. When time and insurance companies permit, if the patient asks for a second opinion, the physician should make it easy for her to obtain pertinent medical records.

Every caregiver, whether they are performing surgery, delivering radiation or chemotherapy, or inserting intravenous lines, should encourage the patient to ask questions. Some doctors fall back too readily on answering questions with scientific jargon or statistics without giving context. Statistics are invaluable—it's impossible to practice medicine without them—but patients who suffer rare complications take little comfort in the statement, "It happens less than 1 percent of the time."

The team approach to breast cancer is a key reason for the improved survival statistics. But even a team approach sometimes has its drawbacks, including poor communication or unnecessarily duplicated tests. Also, a negative or counterproductive attitude by a single person on the team can undo the good work of ten others. It is imperative every caregiver demonstrates patience and tolerance and does what he or she can to instill the patient with courage. Most important, a major part of every caregiver's role is to be an advocate for the patient.

What People Can Do for Themselves

Early detection is the sine qua non of breast cancer treatment. Patients diagnosed early tend to have better survival and cure rates. While there is some give-and-take about the value of regular self-breast examinations, this is indisputably how many patients detect their own cancer. An experienced physician or nurse should educate women on the proper technique and timing of self-examination. Along with self-exam, women should learn breast cancer signs and symptoms, in addition to lumps. Skin changes, unusual breast thickening, nipple discharge, and breast pain can all persist for a long time before the patient brings them to the doctor's attention.

Mammography (imaging) is the cornerstone of early detection, an essential aspect of contemporary public health. Unfortunately, in many parts of the country, mammography services are disappearing. There are fewer imaging machines and fewer doctors to interpret them because mammography is a frequent source of litigation and not always a high-profit area. (Sadly, some in the insurance and medical industry have lost their way in pursuit of profit at the expense of patients.) The good news is that despite some controversy, there is strong consensus that screening through imaging saves lives. Moreover, better and more sophisticated imaging techniques are being developed that will only enhance detection. Be an advocate for more screening mammography programs through your job or place of worship.

Another emerging area of research and treatment where women can take an active role is in the genetics of breast cancer. Women in certain high-risk categories and those with a strong family history of breast cancer are candidates for genetic profiling. In certain cases, the genetic profile suggests the best approach is prophylactic mastectomy. This is an area women should discuss with their doctors to see whether they are candidates for risk assessment and genetic evaluation.

In terms of prevention, much remains to be learned. There are indications that moderate exercise, avoiding obesity, and minimizing alcohol intake may all play a role in lowering the risk of breast cancer.

What You Can Do for Family, Friends, or Acquaintances with Breast Cancer

Become part of their support system in any way possible. Don't avoid them or rationalize "it's better if I don't say anything." In fact small gestures like a phone call, a card, or a pleasant remark mean a lot to the patient. After surgery, tests, and chemotherapy are completed, volunteer to transport the patient to and from the hospital, offer to help with carpooling and caring for kids after school, and provide meals for them and their family. Chemotherapy may only take a few hours, but between travel and the medication side effects, it's usually an all-day event. Patients need help. Coworkers and bosses can be of assistance in adjusting patients' workloads and providing flexibility with work schedules.

Heroes and Gratitude

A word on heroes: While not all patients are candidates for breast cancer studies, a debt of gratitude is owed to those who have participated in studies for most of our advances in the field. They are true unsung heroes of medicine. Demonstrate your gratitude by donating in some way, either money or time, to a breast cancer–related charity.

As devastating as a diagnosis of breast cancer can be, it offers a new perspective on life; it is not all sadness. Patients, family, and friends can have many good moments during the course of the disease. Often they tell jokes together and experience a spirit of camaraderie they might otherwise not have known. Resist any urge to blame yourself for the disease. Remember, some things that happen cannot be prevented. (The two most important breast cancer risk factors, age and family history, are both beyond the power to control.) With the current progress in research and treatment, there is every reason to believe the prognosis for all patients will continue to improve. Finally, keep in mind the things that are truly important—your health and that of your family and friends.

5

ACHING FOR SOME UNDIVIDED MEDICAL ATTENTION

I know I've made some very poor decisions recently,
but I can give you my complete assurance that my work will be back
to normal. I've still got the greatest enthusiasm and confidence
in the mission. And I want to help you.

—HAL 9000 IN *2001: A SPACE ODYSSEY*

I N STANLEY KUBRICK'S classic film *2001: A Space Odyssey*, the survival of astronauts on a space mission depends on a computer, the infallible HAL 9000. HAL relates to the crew in human fashion and keeps them safe until the chilling climax when he decides to engineer their murders by sabotaging the ship's life-support systems. It is the quintessential depiction of the erosion of trust between man and machine.

The medical profession currently faces the same existential crisis. Since being introduced into hospitals, computers have advanced medical care tremendously, but now they represent a serious threat to depersonalize the patient. According to a study in the *Journal of General Internal Medicine*, doctors in training currently spend only 12 percent of their time in direct patient care compared with 40 percent of time spent in front of computers. Moreover, this trend of reduced interaction with patients is growing worse.

It would be tempting to ascribe this development, like so much else in our contemporary culture, to a generational shift in attitudes. As one medical resident told the *New York Times*, "My generation is different because we can't have the same relationships with patients as you did. We just don't have the time."

A nice, facile explanation, but this problem is hardly confined to young trainees. Virtually every attending physician I speak to, including some in their seventies, describes the unsettling number of hours they must spend in front of the computer at the expense of time with the patient.

Nor is this development limited to physicians. Today's modern hospital furnishes nurses with portable computers to enter patient data, write notes, and scan medications. Presumably more efficient, but unquestionably less personal. Nurses, like their physician counterparts, have become more high tech, less high touch.

The resident who spoke to the *New York Times* unwittingly fails to appreciate the twofold problem the current situation presents. First, to become proficient a doctor or nurse must train all five of their senses, which the computer discourages. One must learn to observe by actually looking at the patient. Likewise, learning to talk to the patient, what to ask, as well as when and how, cannot be replicated by a software template of questions.

Hearing is also a skill that must be cultivated—it's more than just listening to a stethoscope (or today an ultrasound); it's listening to what the patient has to say. Touch is important, everything from taking the pulse to palpating masses. And smell can be a means of diagnosis; there are even diseases that can be diagnosed the moment you walk into a patient's room. Staring at a computer screen and tapping on a keyboard might approach but will never reproduce all these things.

But even more significant than acquiring technical proficiency is establishing human contact. The essence of the medical profession is showing patients you really care by creating a personal bond—the manner in which you talk to them, listen to them, and touch them sympathetically and make eye contact. (Tellingly, in *2001: A Space Odyssey*, HAL's lack of human emotion was portrayed by its electronic laser eye, which gave the astronauts nothing to make eye contact with.) No one expressed the essential nature of human contact better than Sir William Osler, considered the preeminent clinician of the twentieth century, who advised the young doctor, "Care more for the individual patient than for the special features of the disease. . . . Put yourself in his place. . . . The kindly word, the cheerful greeting, the sympathetic look—these the patient understands."

Contrast the twentieth-century Oslerian philosophy with the twenty-first-century philosophy expressed by former secretary of health and human services Kathleen Sebelius. In 2010 in *Kaiser Health News*, she wrote, "Over the last 30 years, we've watched information technology revolutionize industry after industry, dramatically improving the customer experience and driving down costs. Today, in almost every other sector besides health, electronic information exchange is the way we do business. A cashier scans a bar code to add up our grocery bill. We check our bank balance and take out cash with a debit card that works in any ATM."

This analogy betrays a fundamental misunderstanding of the art of medicine in any century. Grocery bar codes and ATMs are efficient, albeit depersonalizing examples of technology affecting our lives. But the ideal goal of medical care is to be able to spend more, not less, time with and attention on patients.

Bedside manner is on its deathbed. It can be saved only if the medical community, the tech community, and the government address the proper use and abuse of computers in medicine. The alternative is that in the future patients will be citizens of a dystopian brave new world where anyone may be able to see the doctor, but the doctor won't be looking at them.

6

REPORTING SCIENCE
WITHOUT THE DRAMA

News Items: 25,000 U.S. DEATHS LINKED TO SUGARY DRINKS.
1 IN 10 U.S. DEATHS BLAMED ON SALT.

DRAMATIC HEADLINES, but questionable science. As with other media science coverage, the response left much to be desired. Researchers' findings are often misinterpreted. That's in part due to conclusions that journalists routinely draw but that tend to short-circuit full analysis. The following are all common pitfalls:

The simpler the association, the better. The assertion that twenty-five thousand deaths are annually linked to excess sugar intake is an example of an overly simplistic conclusion attributed to cause and effect. This ignores a host of complicating variables that confound the relationship between diet and mortality (other diseases, genetics, alcohol, tobacco). Even the well-established but incompletely understood association between tobacco and lung cancer is not direct cause and effect; many smokers do not develop cancer, and some nonsmokers do. Despite the facile headlines, cause-effect relations are almost never clear-cut.

Reporting abstracts rather than peer-reviewed studies. Both the salt study and soft drink study are abstracts—preliminary reports that journals and professional societies introduce before peer review. The findings of an abstract have not been subjected to rigorous outside analysis. Publicizing abstracts conveys undue importance before the work has undergone scientific scrutiny. An abstract is to a finished study what a screenplay is to a movie—an essential first step that sometimes yields a finished product, even an occasional blockbuster, but often winds up on the shelf.

The allure of large, round numbers. In 2016 the city of Chicago estimated the attendance along the parade route and at the Grant Park rally for the Chicago Cubs' first championship in over one hundred years was about five million people. The actual number cannot be counted, and reliable estimates require considerable time, effort, and expense. Consequently, a large, round number, accurate or not, is published. A ready example is the widely cited figure, albeit with a shaky foundation, of how hospital errors are responsible for one hundred thousand deaths annually. Originally derived from a 1999 Institute of Medicine estimate, rather than direct observation, the published number was actually a range of forty-four thousand to ninety-eight thousand. The large, round number entered the public domain when sources simply accepted the higher estimate and rounded up, even though the actual figure is unknown and may be far less—closer to or perhaps even below the lower limit of forty-four thousand.

Academic imprimatur. Studies done at prominent research centers generally receive greater attention than those from less prestigious ones. This is expected—Harvard has more experienced researchers, and more research dollars, than Southwest Technical State. However, Harvard research is not intrinsically more valid. This is fallacy of authority—a Harvard study receives more publicity and less scrutiny.

Respected journal. Authority fallacy also occurs because journalists are loath to dissect studies from prestigious journals. In 2006 the *Lancet*, one of the world's top medical journals, published a Johns Hopkins study indicating an excess of six hundred thousand civilian deaths in the first three years of the Iraq War, a finding that seemed implausible on its face. The high death rate meant over five hundred more civilians died each day during the war than before it, a fact that could not be confirmed independently by either the United Nations or the Iraqi government. Widespread, unquestioning television and newspaper coverage of the controversial figures followed, in large measure due to publication in the *Lancet*. However, there was little press follow-up of subsequent analyses by other researchers demonstrating important methodological flaws and ethical questions in the original study. Their research suggested the first study may have overstated civilian casualties by several hundred thousand.

Studies from prestigious-sounding organizations. Reporters gravitate toward studies from "institutes," "foundations," and "schools of public health policy." While these studies are quite often reliable and well done, there is an inherent danger that many of these organizations have a political agenda, whether liberal or conservative, which could be reflected in their work. Individuals who join these organizations may perform research that promotes, either consciously or unconsciously, the organization's biases.

A persuasive spokesperson. Think of it as the Walter Cronkite effect. The authors of a study may dispatch a spokesperson, usually an articulate, knowledgeable researcher, to enhance the study's credibility with the press. Journalists, often with little scientific background, are unwilling or unable to make appropriate inquiries about the study's findings. In this way a study's flaws can easily remain undiscovered.

Publication bias toward positive effects. In reporting scientific studies, the media are prone to cherry-picking—that is, publishing studies that have successful outcomes or suggest an actual effect (such as salt consumption causing death). Scientific journals often exhibit the same bias. In 1991 Canadian researchers analyzed how North American newspapers approached two studies on the association of radiation and cancer, one showing a positive association, the other failing to find one. They concluded, "The number, length and quality of newspaper reports on the positive study were greater than news reports on the negative study, which suggests a bias against news reports of studies showing no effects or no adverse effects."

Do any of these factors by themselves mean media reports about science are necessarily wrong? No, but science is inherently complex, and media coverage often proves Oscar Wilde's observation that the truth is rarely pure and never simple.

7

DR. OZ, HEAL THYSELF, AND "BROADCAST DOCTORS" ON TV

Medicine grounds me, it centers me,
that's why I continue to do it.

—DR. MEHMET OZ

HAS DR. OZ JUMPED THE SHARK? With millions of television viewers and disciples, he is unquestionably the most popular physician in the United States, if not the world. But because his commentaries have begun deviating from traditional medical advice into the realm of unproven natural medicines, nostrums, and occasionally even further into homeopathy and faith healing, that hard-earned popularity has come at a cost to his reputation, especially in the medical community. It says much about medicine on television.

For nearly thirty years, Dr. Oz has been a well-respected cardiac surgeon at one of the country's top medical centers. He has a smooth, poised demeanor on television. Yet in 2014 during his appearance to testify before the Senate Commerce Committee about his testimonials of untested weight loss drugs, he came off looking more like a flustered criminal underboss than a confident surgeon who has deftly operated on hundreds of human hearts.

Much of the advice Dr. Oz dispenses on his television show and his website is grounded in solid science, and his unpretentious approach is immensely popular with the general public. But at virtually every medical center I have visited recently, I notice him being roundly criticized by doctors for his forays into alternative medicine and his increasingly nonscientific approach. No doubt some of this is based on jealousy; some of those doctors would love the exposure and fame he has. But this does not explain it completely. Much of the criticism is legitimate and is getting louder.

Dr. David Gorski, an MD/PhD who is a surgical oncologist in Detroit and the managing editor of the medical blog *Science-Based Medicine*, has been especially critical of Dr. Oz in his blog. He writes, "I keep hoping that someday he'll have an epiphany and realize he is no longer a scientist. Worse, he is no longer a responsible doctor. Instead, he's become an enabler and cheerleader, either wittingly or unwittingly, for quackery."

Several years ago, Benjamin Mazer, a medical student at the University of Rochester, began a public campaign against Dr. Oz. He requested state and national medical societies scrutinize Dr. Oz's advice more closely. He told the website Vox,

Dr. Oz has something like 4-million viewers a day. The average physician doesn't see a million patients in their lifetime. That's why organized medicine should be taking action. . . . I'm definitely not the only one. This issue was brought up by a number of physicians I worked with during my family medicine clerkship. We had all of this first-hand experience with patients who really liked his show and trusted him quite a bit. [Dr. Oz] would give advice that was really not great or it had no medical basis. It might sound harmless when you talk about things like herbal pills or supplements. But when the physicians' advice conflicted with Oz, the patients would believe Oz. . . . Many patients trusted Dr. Oz more than their own family doctors and this conflict hurt the doctor-patient relationship. The trust people are placing with Dr. Oz—when their family physicians even nicely try to contradict him—disrupts their relationship.

Long before Dr. Oz, reality television, and the current glut of TV shows featuring doctors and nurses something of a bright line existed between show business and medicine. Your TV might feature fictional heroes—Ben Casey, Dr. Kildare, or Hawkeye and Trapper John—but real physicians rarely went on television. Ironically, among the only times in the early days of television that actual doctors were mentioned were in cigarette endorsements.

That was then, but now the bright line has vanished. There is no longer any need for disclaimers. Today television loves medicine, with fictional doctors and nurses in situation comedies, detective dramas, and soap operas. Meanwhile real doctors are medical reporters, talk-show guests, and infomercial hosts touting pharmaceuticals and hospitals.

In a well-publicized incident on his syndicated TV show in 2011, Dr. Oz released research showing that some brands of apple juice contained unacceptable levels of arsenic. This drew the ire of the Food and Drug Administration (FDA), which roundly criticized Dr. Oz and reasserted its findings that apple juice is safe to drink.

Dr. Oz, however well intentioned, left himself open to criticism on several points. His research failed to distinguish between toxic and naturally occurring arsenic, the latter widely believed to be harmless. He failed to repeat his studies in a second lab to reconfirm the disturbing results, which would be the logical next step of scientific analysis. Finally, he avoided the question of whether any children had actually suffered arsenic toxicity. Quite to the contrary, he reassured viewers they could continue to let their children drink apple juice, rather surprising advice in the face of what he believed were toxic arsenic levels.

Nevertheless, Dr. Oz deserves credit for demanding accountability from the FDA. He rightfully asked the FDA to be more transparent in its analysis of apple juice and, by extension, in its entire process of food testing. Transparency has been an issue for the FDA in the past, and thanks to Dr. Oz the agency issued new rules on arsenic levels in apple juice to avoid a public health scare.

The question of apple juice toxicity demonstrates the mixed blessing in the marriage between medicine and show business. Besides raising the public health consciousness, television medicine creates more educated consumers. People can now receive what amounts to a near equivalent of a premedical education served up on television. Does this plethora of diagnoses, surgery, and drugs on the tube serve the public well?

In many respects, yes. Many patients receive screening and therapy more promptly than in the past, they ask better questions when being examined, and occasionally they are able to alert the doctor to conditions and treatments the doctor may not have considered. Show business can, and occasionally does, save lives.

But the benefit is not unalloyed. The flip side is that television can mislead the public (witness the FDA brickbats, legitimate or not, thrown at Dr. Oz). There is a mutual exploitation between television and medicine. Television, in its eternal quest for ratings, invariably trolls for what's new, exciting, and trendy. This often distorts reality in a manner antithetical to the nature of medicine, where knowledge is often accrued gradually and it often takes years to prove a treatment's effectiveness or danger.

But the exploitation is not all one-sided. Health care is also big business. There are hucksters in the pharmaceutical and hospital industries who understand the immense sales potential of television and doctors who, for reasons of greed or vanity, willingly cozy up to the camera. They may exaggerate the benefits or underplay the risks of pharmaceuticals and surgeries. Every medication or surgical procedure carries some risk, and by the same token, any infomercial, press release, or celebrity endorsement may carry a hidden agenda or misrepresentation.

To a certain extent, the problem is that blurred boundary between medicine and show business. In the 1980s, a cough syrup commercial featured a soap opera actor intoning that now oft-parodied phrase, "I'm not a doctor, but I play one on TV." That disclaimer was meant to prevent the public from getting the impression they were watching a physician's endorsement. But television, with its insatiable appetite for content good and bad, has since co-opted the medical profession, with Dr. Oz as the poster boy.

Moreover, like every successful long-running television show, Dr. Oz ultimately faces the same problem—diminishing quality. (The term *jump the shark* came from the popular 1970s sitcom *Happy Days*. After so many years on the air, it became obvious the show had exceeded its shelf life when Fonzie, the show's star, waterskied over a man-eating shark.)

Dr. Oz has done hundreds of hours of shows, and there are, after all, only so many ways to dispense reliable advice about scientific medicine and healthy living. Eventually his show must explore the neighborhood where snake oil salesmen reside, and avoiding that neighborhood becomes progressively harder with another show coming up soon.

There is plenty to be learned about your health from television. But it is not to be confused with reality. Find a trusted physician or health care provider and discuss everything you hear about medicine on television. That's the best way to get the straight story on treatments that can save your life—and allow you to avoid those that might harm you. It also keeps your doctors on their toes. Keep in mind that when you watch medicine or medical drama on-screen, show business wants to portray real life, but it is perfectly willing to sacrifice real life for the sake of entertainment. Caveat emptor.

As for Dr. Oz, when he is at his best, he has helped countless people with his medical guidance. He has undoubtedly saved many lives and deserves appropriate credit for that. He remains a brilliant physician and, according to those who work with him, a superb surgeon. He is certainly without peer as a medical communicator. But when he looks in the mirror these days, does Dr. Oz ask himself the eternal biblical question, "For what shall it profit a man, if he shall gain the whole world, and lose his own soul?"

8

PHYSICIAN-JOURNALISTS

The first duty of the physician is to educate the masses.
—Sir William Osler, MD

MEDICAL STORIES—whether the subject is epidemic outbreaks, celebrity deaths, or the victims of distant wars and disasters—are surefire attention getters. For that reason, most major news organization have a physician-journalist on staff, and some are household names, such as CNN's Sanjay Gupta, a neurosurgeon, and Richard Besser, a pediatric infectious disease specialist who in 2017 left his position as ABC chief health and medicine editor to become president and CEO of the Robert Wood Johnson Foundation. But when physician-journalists report medical stories, are they primarily reporters or doctors? Can they be both at the same time?

These ethical questions arose when Dr. Gupta, covering a 2015 earthquake as part of the CNN news team in Nepal, performed an emergency neurosurgical procedure on an eight-year-old girl and then performed brief cardiopulmonary resuscitation on a second patient in a rescue helicopter.

Both episodes were shown to audiences on television. At first blush is there anything wrong with showing audiences compelling footage of Dr. Gupta employing his medical skills to help save lives?

There are two problems, one medical and the other journalistic. From a medical standpoint, showing the patients being treated on international television is technically a violation of medical confidentiality. In neither case was it likely Dr. Gupta obtained consent for filming the patients. According to the Hippocratic oath, "Whatever I see or hear in the lives of my patients, whether in connection with my professional practice or not, which ought not to be spoken of outside, I will keep secret, as considering all such things to be private." The principle of medical confidentiality doesn't change, even if television wasn't referred to in the ancient Greek oath.

The second problem is one all journalists, especially those on television, face when covering a story. At what point does the reporter, instead of the subject, become part of the story or even the primary focus of the story? The drama of treating a patient on television is an ever-present temptation for the reporter or the network to use as a promotional vehicle, and the patient becomes nothing more than a prop being exploited ("Breaking news: Tune in at ten to see Dr. Gupta perform brain surgery!"). In the face of such self-promotion, any pretense of objectivity is lost. This doesn't mean that an audience can't see a doctor treating a patient or performing surgery. It means the doctor who is treating the patient should not be the same one who reports the story.

In Nepal Dr. Gupta's primary job was as a reporter, to describe conditions in the area ravaged by the earthquake. If patients needed emergency medical care that only Dr. Gupta was available to render, his obligation became to treat the patients, and at that point, he gave up being a reporter. But his crew should have turned off their cameras and not aired the footage of the treatment.

The same issues arose during the 2010 earthquake in Haiti when Dr. Gupta examined and treated a baby with head trauma on camera, and Dr. Besser was filmed caring for a pregnant Haitian woman in labor. In those situations, both doctors came perilously close to becoming the subject of the stories at the expense of patients in extremis.

Following the Haiti earthquake, Tom Linden, a physician and professor of medical journalism in the School of Journalism and Mass Communication at the University of North Carolina, proposed guidelines for physician-journalists. His first rule was that when there is no alternative in a life-threatening medical emergency, physician-journalists should act as doctors and treat the patient; their responsibility as reporters is secondary. When they do treat a patient, it should not be featured on television. In all situations any identifiable patient should give consent before appearing on television (and in the case of children, consent should be obtained from a parent or guardian). And there is a general presumption that any treatment by the physician should never be contingent on having the person consent to being on television.

Dr. Linden's rules are a sensible attempt to establish boundaries between the two roles of physician-journalists. Sometimes the line between those roles is not a bright one, and it is not always easy to see. In this respect, I am not beyond reproach. I regret I may have occasionally crossed the line at a patient's expense in my writings and interviews. It is admittedly difficult to maintain the boundaries between the role as a physician and as a journalist. But it is incumbent on physician-journalists to recognize how important the separation is. Otherwise they put at risk their two most valuable assets—their integrity as physicians and their credibility as journalists.

II

HEROES AND VILLAINS

9

IN PRAISE OF FIRST-RATE MEDICINE

At a given instant everything the surgeon knows suddenly becomes
important to the solution of the problem. You can't do it an hour
later, or tomorrow. Nor can you go to the library and look it up.

—JOHN KIRKLIN, MD

L ET US NOW PRAISE FAMOUS MEN AND WOMEN: the paramedics
and medical professionals who performed heroically after the 2013
Boston Marathon bombings. Despite the efforts of cold-blooded killers
who constructed antipersonnel devices packed with ball bearings and nails
designed for maximum lethality, there were only three deaths from the
bombings among more than 260 victims. That is amazing.

How did the Boston medical community achieve such remarkable
results? It began with the coordination between first responders and hospitals, working with lessons learned from military medicine. The treatment
of hemorrhage and shock has been refined incrementally from World War

II to Korea, Vietnam, and finally the Gulf Wars. Military surgeons have observed that rather than immediate wound repair in the field, more lives are saved by emphasizing rapid control of bleeding at the site followed by stabilization and transport for definitive surgery. This was the primary focus at the marathon site.

Next, the triage at the medical centers was excellent. It is an underappreciated skill to rapidly sort out the seriously wounded requiring immediate surgery from those who need urgent but nonsurgical attention from the less urgent walking wounded. The doctors and nurses in the emergency departments performing triage must think fast and use quick judgment; errors at that stage are frequently fatal. When the marathon casualties arrived, the medical teams performed superbly.

The small number of deaths also speaks to the quality of surgery performed on those who survived the explosions. In the case of bombs like those detonated at the Boston Marathon, blast injuries are a frightening amalgam of blunt and penetrating trauma, burns, and wounds from shrapnel composed of dirt, metal, nails, and ball bearings, along with clothing and bone (sometimes from other victims). The three unfortunate marathon fatalities were in the early period, and the fact that the subsequent fatality count did not rise means there were no delayed, fatal surgical misadventures or infections. Remember, all this occurred amid the confusion of hospital mass disaster responses.

Having participated in and coordinated hospital mass disaster responses in Chicago, I can testify that the best of these are often little more than controlled chaos. It is always extremely difficult to account for large numbers of unanticipated admissions. Many victims are admitted without identification, and because of injuries are unable to identify themselves. Patient charts often get misplaced, and keeping track of everyone involved is difficult. (One of the young women who died in the marathon bombing was initially misidentified to her family as being alive.) These problems become exponentially more difficult with investigating law enforcement officials, hordes of reporters, worried family members, and curious onlookers besieging the hospital.

Finally, no experienced medical professional with humility would discount the role of serendipity when lives are saved. Since the marathon is a significant civic event in Boston, there were extra first aid stations, less vehicular traffic, and more medical personnel available than on a normal day. Most of the victims were young and thus better able to withstand serious injuries than those at the extremes of age. Finally, the nature of the explosions was such that the force was concentrated low to the ground. The blast injuries were primarily to lower extremities, devastating to be sure but not as prone to inflicting life-threatening damage as those to the torso, chest, or head.

Unfortunately, the blast injuries to the lower extremities resulted in extensive limb damage, in many cases necessitating amputation. Here again the knowledge gained and techniques perfected in battlefield care have spread to civilian medicine. Limb injury and amputation have been one of the most common results of the use of the improvised explosive device (IED) by the enemy in Iraq and Afghanistan. However, the same human ingenuity that creates weapons of combat and the capacity to kill also discovers ways to heal and save lives. Now amputees can be fitted with state-of-the-art prosthetics made from high-tech plastics and metal alloys. Using microprocessors and hydraulics, these sophisticated prosthetics employ sensors that react to electronic impulses from intact muscles. One day soon, amputees may be able to move a prosthetic limb simply by concentrating on the movements.

To paraphrase Winston Churchill, for the medical victims of the marathon bombing, this is not the end or even the beginning of the end, merely the end of the beginning. They and their families will forever live with devastating physical damage and psychological trauma. As a society, we must offer these people our ongoing care, compassion, counseling, opportunities for employment, and most important our understanding. For the first responders and medical personnel who did such a magnificent job treating the casualties on Patriots' Day, the appreciation and gratitude owed to them is immeasurable.

10

THE GHOSTS OF COOK COUNTY

The lawn
Is pressed by unseen feet, and ghosts return
Gently at twilight, gently go at dawn,
The sad intangible who grieve and yearn. . . .

—T. S. ELIOT

THE OLD COOK COUNTY HOSPITAL BUILDING, built in 1914, stands partially torn down, but there are plans to reconfigure it for office and residential use sometime in the future. I worked there for three decades and knew people who worked there as far back as the 1930s. I took the news of the new plans with mixed emotions—any plan to revitalize the beautiful facade is better than how it sits now amid garbage, weeds, and graffiti.

But something bothered me. While there are plans for a hotel, shops, and apartments, no provisions have been made for the thousands of ghosts living there. Many of those ghosts of the past I knew personally; others I learned about from my predecessors. They all exist as memories and markers of a crucial Chicago institution.

The emaciated old men dying of tuberculosis. The emaciated young men dying of AIDS. The young women who died of uterine infections after illegal abortions. The young unwed mothers, barely out of grade school. The heroin addicts dying of overdoses. The patients from the Madison Street flophouses who went into delirium tremens when they couldn't buy alcohol.

The trauma patients with the type of wounds that doctors rarely saw outside the battlefield. The patients from foreign countries with exotic infections none of us had seen before. The patients who died of heat stroke when there was no air-conditioning on the open wards and the windows could not be opened. The people who wanted to kill themselves by jumping out of the building. The few who succeeded.

The doctors who saved patients with their brilliance and their daring. The doctors who killed patients with their arrogance and stupidity. The physicians who became nationally renowned and the ones who took kickbacks. The surgeons who invented new surgical techniques and the ones who operated drunk. The doctor who invented the blood bank and the doctors who charged patients for blood transfusions. The doctors who smoked cigarettes while they made rounds on the large, open wards. The intern who was stabbed to death by a patient.

The nurses who selflessly volunteered to come in whenever there was an emergency. The nurses who were so talented they could place intravenous lines in any patient and the medical students who couldn't put them in anyone. The overworked but always well-intentioned social workers. The unsung patient transporters, the radiology technicians, and the therapists. The electricians, maintenance men, buildings and grounds men, custodians, and cooks. The elevator operators who got Election Day off to get out the vote but kept their jobs even after the elevators became push button.

The staffers who cheated on their overtime. The chaplains. The county board presidents. The security guard who denied a county board president entry to the hospital because he didn't have identification. The crooked politicians—and the occasional honest one. The county commissioners who went to jail. The hospital administrators who were glorified political hacks.

The union stooges and management flunkies. The anarchists, communists, left-wingers, and right-wingers. The doctor who serendipitously discovered the identity of mass murderer Richard Speck when Speck came to the emergency room during a nationwide manhunt. Richard Speck, twenty years later a jailhouse prostitute. The gangbangers, numbers runners, and Syndicate killers. The patients who sold drugs in the stairwells. The hookers who plied their trade in the stairwells. The doctors on call who made love with nurses in vacant offices at night.

The brave policemen who died in the trauma unit, killed in the line of duty. The courageous firemen who died of smoke inhalation and burns. The cops on the take and those who worked covertly for the Outfit. The newspaper and television reporters who came to the hospital but never stayed long enough to get the facts right.

The famous visitors like Princess Diana, Mr. T, Harrison Ford, then state senator Barack Obama, and Dan Rostenkowski—when he was the most powerful man in the US House of Representatives. Linda Darnell, dying in the burn unit twenty years removed from being the most beautiful woman in Hollywood. Major Lance, thirty years after he had the number-one R&B hit in the country.

The forgotten jazz musicians. The Negro League ballplayers who played with Satchel Paige. The babies who grew up to be Harold Washington, Herbie Hancock, Curtis Mayfield, Bernie Mac, and Phil Everly (of the Everly Brothers).

The great-grandmothers. The great-grandchildren. The premature infants who died, never having come off the ventilator. And the ones who miraculously survived to grow up healthy and have families.

Now with the new plan for the building, those ghosts will have to move. For a time, they can reside in my memory and that of those who came before me. But at some unspecified future date, those memories are also scheduled for demolition.

When that happens, where will all those ghosts live?

11

THE MAN WHO SAVED PITCHERS' ARMS

There are a lot of pitchers in baseball who should celebrate his life and what he did for the game of baseball.

—TOMMY JOHN ON DR. FRANK JOBE

DR. FRANK JOBE, a humble but accomplished orthopedic surgeon, died in 2014 at the age of eighty-eight. He salvaged the careers of countless baseball players by pioneering the "Tommy John surgery," a revolutionary elbow ligament repair. He was unquestionably the greatest orthopedic surgeon in professional sports history, the Babe Ruth of the profession. Dr. James Andrews, today's leading sports orthopedic surgeon, said of Jobe in the *Los Angeles Times*, "Without his influence, baseball players' sports-medicine care would probably still be in the Dark Ages."

But Jobe's passing also raises questions about the evolution of medicine since 1974, when he first tried the experimental technique on Tommy John, an injured Los Angeles Dodgers pitcher. Four decades later, in a world where government and corporate bureaucracies strive to minimize practice variations among physicians and "evidence-based guidelines" dictate medical practice, would it be possible for a freethinking medical innovator like Jobe to introduce such a radically new, untested surgical procedure?

The story of the first Tommy John surgery, technically known as ulnar collateral ligament reconstruction, is testimony not only to surgical excellence but also to the ineffable bond between a physician and patient. Jobe was the Dodgers' orthopedist when John, a decent but not great pitcher, felt severe pain in his pitching arm. He suddenly could not deliver a pitch, and Jobe diagnosed an ulnar collateral ligament tear, a career-ending injury.

John, disconsolate at the thought of life without baseball, was not just Jobe's patient but also his friend. He implored the surgeon to try anything that would allow him to pitch again. Sympathetic to his friend's plight, the doctor agreed and considered an operation that had never been tried on a baseball pitcher. Jobe had previously worked with polio patients, for whom surgeons transplanted tendons from other parts of the body to reinforce immobilized limbs. Could a transplanted tendon work on a major league pitcher, for whom the mechanical stress on the elbow is exponentially greater?

Jobe discussed the operation with John, who was willing to try it. He took a tendon from the pitcher's nonpitching arm and wove it tightly through holes drilled in the bone of the injured left elbow. In essence the transplanted tendon from John's nonpitching arm became the new ulnar ligament for his pitching arm. Uncertain of how it would work, Jobe gave John a 1 percent chance of ever pitching again.

Jobe's pessimism turned out to be misplaced. John became a great pitcher with a twenty-six-year career, one of the longest in major league history. He won more games after his surgery than before. Buoyed by its success, Jobe taught the procedure to other orthopedic surgeons. Those surgeons have gone on to perform the operation on more than one thousand major leaguers, only a fraction of the thousands of minor leaguers, college and high school players, and other athletes who have had Tommy

John surgery. Of particular note, David Wells had the operation as a minor leaguer in 1985 and pitched a perfect game for the New York Yankees in 1998.

In medicine, like all else, timing is everything. Eight years before Jobe operated on John, another Dodger left-hander was forced to retire with the same injury at the height of his career. One can only speculate what might have been had Jobe committed earlier to do the procedure on the greatest of them all, Sandy Koufax.

Today Jobe and John are both honored in each other's profession. John's name is ubiquitous in the orthopedic medical literature for the eponymous surgery, and Jobe was honored in a special contributors' wing in the Baseball Hall of Fame. But would it be possible for Jobe to introduce the Tommy John surgery today? Corporatization and the government have drastically diminished the role of the individual physician. New barriers have been constructed between patient and physician.

Consider this: Would hospital administrators or government watchdogs prevent Jobe from performing this new operation because it is not approved by the medical establishment that sets the rules? Would the profession dissuade Jobe from helping John without randomized controlled studies that take years to perform? Would medical center institutional review boards permit Jobe to operate? Would lawyer-drafted, unreadable twenty-page informed consent forms scare off John? Would insurance companies authorize payment for such an experimental procedure in future patients?

In 1974, before persuading Jobe to try surgery, a desperate Tommy John considered consulting a knuckleball specialist to teach him that difficult pitch, which puts little stress on the elbow. Fortunately, John was a friend of a loyal, talented, and resourceful physician who was brave enough to challenge the medical orthodoxy and health care system of the day. It might happen the same way today, but just maybe today John would be told to learn to throw a knuckleball. And the next Frank Jobe would remain unknown.

12

THE WOMAN WHO PROTECTED US

They were writing letters and telephoning.
They were very anxious to get their product on the market.
It had been very successful in other countries and they felt there
would be a big market in this country. Then quite suddenly,
the news came from Europe about the deformities.

—FRANCES KELSEY, MD, ON RICHARDSON-MERRELL'S DESIRE
TO MARKET THALIDOMIDE TO PREGNANT WOMEN
IN THE UNITED STATES

N THE LATE 1950s, German scientists developed a "wonder drug" for women that was supposed to alleviate the morning sickness, insomnia, and headaches of pregnancy. German studies touted the medication as safe, and it was distributed widely throughout Europe. The drug, thalidomide, became an immediate international success, and there was a move to bring it quickly to the lucrative American market. That would have happened had it not been for one physician working for the Food and Drug Administration (FDA), a brave woman largely forgotten today, named Dr. Frances Kelsey.

She was suspicious of the haphazard European testing and resisted pressure for approval from the drug company, as well as from her superiors at the FDA. With only a month on the job at the time, her position at the FDA was already tenuous. However, with good science on her side, she stood fast against approval until further testing could prove thalidomide was safe to fetuses.

In 1961, before American approval was obtained, her diligence was vindicated when the drug was shown to be linked to birth defects. Worldwide more than ten thousand "thalidomide babies" suffered missing or deformed arms and legs. Because thalidomide was never approved for use in the United States, fewer than fifty of those infants were born here. Kelsey single-handedly prevented a nationwide tragedy, provided a model for effective government drug regulation, and changed the culture and mission of the FDA.

Over a half century ago, in a 1962 White House ceremony, President John F. Kennedy awarded Dr. Kelsey the highest honor an American civilian can receive, the President's Award for Distinguished Federal Civilian Service. She was only the second woman to receive the award, and she was hailed publicly by President Kennedy for her valor. After she retired, the FDA named an award in her honor "to celebrate courage and decision-making." She should go down as one of the great physicians and true heroes of twentieth-century American medicine.

There is a teachable moment here. A fungal meningitis outbreak that swept the country in 2012 and caused at least sixty-four deaths was linked to spinal injections of a contaminated steroid. The Massachusetts company that prepared the contaminated steroid solution, the New England Compounding Center (NECC), engaged in a practice known as "drug compounding": a pharmacy makes an individualized preparation of an approved medication for a specific patient according to a physician's instructions. Drug compounding can be helpful to patients requiring precisely tailored medications, and compounding pharmacies can often supply them easier and more cheaply than major drug manufacturers. However, the FDA does not regulate drug compounding. In the NECC case, the approved medication for back injections was suspected of being contaminated with fungus during the compounding process. Estimates are that as many as fourteen thousand patients nationwide received potentially tainted drugs, and more than seven hundred developed meningitis.

Compounding has had problems before. The Institute for Safe Medication Practice has documented twenty-two significant drug compounding errors since 1990, involving seventy-one different drugs and more than two hundred adverse events. The NECC manufacturing disaster was the worst in the United States since 1937, when a company inadvertently mixed an antibiotic with antifreeze, killing more than one hundred people. Federal drug regulation demands a delicate balance.

Overregulation can drive up the cost of drugs and create bottlenecks to useful medications reaching the public; this was a problem in the 1980s during the early years of the AIDS epidemic. Amid widespread criticism, the FDA eventually relaxed its standards to open the drug pipeline to effective AIDS medications. However, when regulators pay too little attention, the system is left open to serious medical tragedies such as the thalidomide episode and the fungal meningitis outbreak.

That is why the medical community, largely silent on the issue until now, must demand stricter FDA oversight of the drug-compounding process. It's time to recall the heroism of Dr. Frances Kelsey, the woman who saved the nation from a medical disaster decades ago with her attention to the importance of drug testing and oversight.

13

NEEDLES TO SAY

The reward for work well done is the opportunity to do more.

—JONAS SALK

I N THE EARLY 1950s, a polio epidemic ravaged North America and Europe. In circumstances largely forgotten today, people avoided drinking fountains, swimming pools, and movie theaters. Summer camps and schools were closed, and even with these measures, thousands caught the disease and died or were permanently disabled. Many spent months in iron lungs separated from friends and family.

Then in 1955, physician-researcher Jonas Salk and his team developed a successful polio vaccine, and Salk was hailed as a national hero. Thousands of lives were saved, and thousands more were spared the debilitating effects of polio. Salk was on the cover of *Time* magazine—in the days when that was a true accomplishment, not a vacuous celebration of celebrity. Interviewed on the famous television program *See It Now* by Edward R. Murrow, Salk was asked, "Who owns the patent on this vaccine?" Dr. Salk replied, "Well, the people, I would say. There is no patent. Could you patent the sun?"

It was certainly a different era, but that story has a special resonance in my family. At the same time Salk was becoming a household name, my father, also a doctor, developed a far less dramatic medical innovation but one that nonetheless saved its small share of lives.

At Cook County Hospital, my father had gained a reputation as an expert clinician and teacher. Doctors in those days spent many more hours in the hospital than they do now, and my father cultivated a hobby: refining ordinary medical instruments, making them easier for doctors and nurses to use. My father would tinker with the EKG machines and lab equipment, always looking for a way to improve them. One of his contemporaries observed that besides being a good doctor, he was "a clever gadgeteer." In those days, there was no government regulatory scrutiny or review boards; if there were he probably would have taken up contract bridge.

Aware of his reputation, several nephrologists from the University of Chicago came to visit him one day. They were the local experts at a new technique—diagnosing and treating kidney diseases by doing kidney biopsies. This involved inserting a needle into the kidney, cutting a small sample of tissue, and extracting it to be studied later under the microscope. Routine today, it was all very high tech at the time. But the technique had run into a problem—before World War II, two men, Vim and Silverman, had devised a crude biopsy needle, which was still employed, and their needle often failed to capture a sufficient amount of tissue to study.

Undaunted, my father saw no difficulty. Within a short time, he modified the bevel on the needle, and the new tool became known as the Franklin modification of the Vim-Silverman needle or simply the Franklin needle. It was an immediate success. Sometime later a leading nephrology journal wrote, "The modification of the needle by Dr. Murray Franklin of Cook County Hospital in Chicago was minor but crucial. . . . For 15 years that was the standard renal biopsy needle used worldwide."

The elated nephrologists now did biopsies and published papers, eventually making Chicago the center of kidney biopsies and renal pathology in the world. Other medical centers quickly picked up on it. A nephrologist pioneering kidney biopsies at Vanderbilt University donated one of the first Franklin needles used there to the Smithsonian Institution's National Museum of History, Medical Sciences Division. My father, barely fazed by these developments, went back to caring for patients and teaching residents.

But the story was just beginning. Cook County Hospital also had a number of world-class gastroenterologists who specialized in liver diseases, and they had started doing liver biopsies to diagnose hepatitis and cirrhosis. They knew my father, who had done his postgraduate research in alcoholic liver disease, and they approached him to see if the Franklin needle would work as well for liver biopsies as it did for kidney biopsies. He told them matter-of-factly that since the liver was a larger, more accessible organ than the kidney, it should work even better on that organ—which is exactly what happened. The Franklin needle also became the standard liver biopsy needle, first in Chicago, then all over the world.

Thousands upon thousands of liver biopsies were done as the Franklin needle became a routine hospital instrument everywhere. It was instrumental to our modern understanding of liver pathology. In the 1960s, ambitious researchers from all over the country even started doing biopsies of the lung with it (although it wasn't as good a tool for lung biopsies). The market for the needle expanded even more when veterinarians started using it to biopsy organs in animals.

By this time, my father had moved on from academic medicine and never personally used the needle again. He rarely gave it a second thought. Growing up, I don't recall ever hearing him mention it. I was vaguely aware of it since my mother occasionally told my sister and me about "the Franklin needle" used in the hospital. My parents' friends, some of whom were physicians, would mention it to us when we were young as something of which to be proud. But it still made little impression on us.

That changed one afternoon when I was in medical school. I was on the wards at Northwestern Memorial Hospital as a junior medical student. My job was basically to follow orders. A classmate and I were sent by the gastroenterologist we were shadowing to bring him a liver biopsy kit with a Franklin needle. At first unaware, it finally dawned on me what he had asked for. Normally students are seen and not heard, but I piped up, "My father invented that needle."

He looked at me skeptically and eyed my name tag (thus confirming my impression that before that moment he hadn't the faintest idea of what my name was—junior medical students, like Rodney Dangerfield, get no respect). After another skeptical moment, he beamed, "Your father is Murray Franklin? This needle revolutionized liver biopsies. You must be rich."

I felt an instant surge of pride that was quickly tempered by a sinking feeling. I certainly wasn't rich, at least not that I was aware of, and suddenly I realized something might be amiss. For some reason, I conjured up the image of all those old blues singers who made classic recordings but made very little money, their profits siphoned off by managers and record companies. Returning to the gastroenterologist, I smiled and let the matter drop. He treated me with greater respect the rest of the month and gave me a better grade than I deserved.

As I progressed in my medical career, I came into contact with more and more specialists who used the needle. I never talked about it, but I realized even small payments to the creator of such a widely used innovation might be substantial. I refrained from asking my father about it for another decade. And I thought of the question Jonas Salk asked Edward R. Murrow. When finally I did ask my father, his response was terse and matter-of-fact: "We didn't patent things like that in those days." I never mentioned it again.

14

AIR-CONDITIONING: A LIFESAVER

The rich get their ice in the summer,
the poor get theirs in the winter.

—LAURA INGALLS WILDER

THE LAST THING in the world I want to do is to get on the wrong side of God, the Catholic Church, or any of my Catholic friends. But I feel compelled to say that Pope Francis, however infallible he might be in matters spiritual, is just plain wrong about air-conditioning.

In his 2015 encyclical, "Laudato Si," the pope wrote, "People may well have a growing ecological sensitivity, but it has not succeeded in changing their harmful habits of consumption, which, rather than decreasing, appear to be growing all the more. A simple example is the increasing use and power of air conditioning. The markets, which immediately benefit from sales, stimulate ever-greater demand. An outsider looking at our world would be amazed at such behavior, which at times appears self-destructive."

Coincidentally, July 2015 marked the twentieth anniversary of the Chicago heat wave that caused nearly eight hundred deaths citywide. The mortality at Cook County Hospital, where I worked, was disproportionately high because many patients were elderly, poor, and, most important, didn't have air-conditioning in their homes.

The majority of deaths during the Chicago heat wave were patients who were already ill, where excessive heat was a major contributing factor. Most patients' cardiovascular systems could not stand the aggravating stress of five days of intense July heat. But two patients in particular stand out in my mind because both of them actually developed severe heatstroke and died while they were inpatients. When they were admitted, their body temperatures were normal, but they died because there was no air-conditioning in the hospital and their body temperatures subsequently climbed to more than 106 degrees.

In 1995 Cook County Hospital occupied the building constructed in 1914 at the corner of Harrison and Wood. (The facade of the partially demolished building still stands.) Other than the operating room, emergency room, intensive care units, and, of course, the administrators' offices, the old building had no air-conditioning. During the heat wave, the general wards were stifling, and conditions for patients were unbearable. There were no private rooms on the wards, and opening what windows could be opened yielded no relief because the recirculated air was so hot.

For several days, patients were continuously exposed to oppressive room temperatures that were often as high or higher than the temperatures outside. It was so bad that it was impossible to tell which patients were running fevers. When the nurses took temperatures, virtually everyone had a temperature of at least 100 degrees.

The two patients who died of heatstroke were elderly, bedridden, and could not dissipate excess body heat and cool themselves by bathing in cold water in the bathrooms as others did. Two other patients developed heatstroke but were transferred to the intensive care unit and survived. Soon afterward portable air conditioners were installed on the wards.

This was something from an earlier era; while dangerous body temperatures can result from medication reactions, no physician or nurse I knew had ever seen a patient already in the hospital develop heatstroke and die. Since today's hospitals, including the rebuilt Cook County Hospital, are air-conditioned, it is unlikely this will ever happen in the absence of a power failure (although a decade later some inpatients at Charity Hospital in New Orleans might have developed heatstroke after Hurricane Katrina knocked out the power).

The role of air-conditioning in preventing heat-related deaths cannot be overestimated. Since 1995, Chicago has had several sweltering summers, but the mortality has not been close to what was seen that July. This is due to greater awareness of the danger of high temperatures and public health measures, including outreach to vulnerable citizens, combined with an effort to provide those at risk with access to cooling centers and air-conditioned buildings. Studies have indicated that mortality during American heat waves has dropped by 80 percent since 1960, with virtually every study concluding the decline in deaths is explained by the adoption of air-conditioning.

In 2015 more than three thousand people died as a result of severe heat waves in Pakistan and on the Indian subcontinent. Virtually all the victims lacked access to reliable electricity and, obviously, air-conditioning. As one study that examined the drop in American heat wave deaths concluded, "Residential air conditioning appears to be the most promising technology to help poor countries mitigate the temperature-related mortality impacts of climate change."

Meanwhile, writer Shubhankar Chhokra pointed out in the blog *Hot Air* that next door to the pope's residence in the air-conditioned Domus Sanctae Marthae is the Vatican Secret Archives, where ancient documents are protected in a temperature-controlled environment. Right next to that is the Sistine Chapel, where the Vatican recently installed a sophisticated air-conditioning system to prevent heat, dust, and carbon dioxide from damaging the priceless frescoes of Michelangelo.

Take note, Pope Francis: such is the revolutionary power of modern air-conditioning. The book of Luke advises, "When you give a banquet, invite the poor, the crippled, the lame, the blind." Today it might have added, "And so they will be safe, take care the banquet hall is air-conditioned in the summertime."

15

FLIGHT 191 ON A SPRING DAY

American 191 Heavy, you want to come back in? What runway?

—LAST GROUND TRANSMISSION FROM
O'HARE CONTROL TOWER TO FLIGHT 191

THE MEMORIAL DAY weekend of 1979 began beautifully, erasing memories of the record snowstorms that had battered Chicago only months before. The mild Lake Michigan breezes, aroma of blossoms, and trees filled with robins stood in contrast to the snows that turned out to be a footnote to world history. (The heavy snows that winter ended the dominance of the Daley Democratic machine and ultimately paved the way for Chicago's first African American mayor, Harold Washington, who in turn became the role model for Barack Obama.)

At O'Hare International Airport, American Airlines Flight 191 was cleared for takeoff, beginning its afternoon flight to Los Angeles. Suddenly, as the massive jet departed the runway, its left engine fell off, disabling critical flight systems. The plane rolled and quickly plummeted to Earth, igniting its full jet-fuel tanks, creating a huge explosion and fireball visible for miles in the azure sky.

On the ground, the grisly inferno resembled a battlefield after a particularly gruesome encounter. Except for 9/11, the crash of Flight 191 remains the worst air disaster in American history—all 271 people on the plane and two people on the ground were killed instantly. Almost all were burned beyond recognition. That afternoon at Cook County Hospital it was shift change when the head nurse was informed the plane had just crashed. A code red—major external disaster—was called. At the time, we were unaware there were no survivors.

As the senior resident in the intensive care unit, along with the trauma and burn teams, I had to coordinate the plan for admitting and caring for crash victims. A quick count of available beds indicated we could take fifty critical patients and another fifty less critical patients. We were told to prepare for ambulances and to mobilize staff immediately.

Fortunately, most of the nurses and respiratory therapists scheduled to leave at shift change voluntarily stayed. That type of selfless response is one of the most gratifying things about working in medicine and typical of how medical personnel respond in emergencies. Everyone went to his or her respective area to ensure there were enough intravenous fluid bags, ventilators, bandages, and other equipment. I rounded up all the available interns. Then there was nothing to do but wait for the ambulances.

Today hospitals have television sets everywhere—patient rooms, waiting areas, cafeterias. Between Twitter and CNN's immediate presence at disasters, everyone is in real-time touch with events. But back then, the only television at County was in the office of an administrator who had left early for the weekend.

While waiting for word of the crash survivors, I felt akin to what I imagine soldiers feel before going into battle—minus the personal danger, of course. A frisson of self-doubt, combined with a touch of frightened exhilaration. What would happen if thirty patients came in immediately? My mind raced. Did we have enough staff? What were they doing at

Rush-Presbyterian and Northwestern Memorial Hospital? Could County handle this?

In less than an hour, the issue became moot. The head nurse announced somberly, "Code red over. No survivors." For a minute, people stared at each other blankly. Even veteran nurses, used to experiencing death, were shocked.

It became a typical Friday night. Overdoses, gunshot victims, drunks.

For me the postscript came two days later when I had to fly to California. By coincidence I was flying American Airlines in the same type of plane as Flight 191. The flight number was close in sequence, perhaps 195 or 197. At the terminal, seeing people reading Sunday newspapers filled with terrible pictures of the 191 crash was quite unsettling. (It was reminiscent of the famous picture of the New York commuter train with every passenger reading the headlines of the JFK assassination.) When we boarded, the pilot announced the flight path would be directly over the still-smoldering crash site. Investigators and emergency vehicles would be easily visible from the plane. To compensate us for having to fly over this horrific scene, the airline offered each passenger a free voucher for a one-way trip anywhere in the United States.

No one looked out the window during takeoff.

16

NEWTOWN PTSD

And the memory dangled over his heart like the sword of Damocles.

—JOSEPH WAMBAUGH, *THE ONION FIELD*

THE AFTERMATH of the 2012 Sandy Hook Elementary School mass shooting irrevocably altered the lives of the victims' families. Now the first responders are also suffering profound repercussions. One Newtown police officer has been diagnosed with post-traumatic stress disorder (PTSD); other cases are anticipated. As a union lawyer for the police told the *New York Times*, "Our concern from the beginning has been the effects of PTSD. We estimate it is probably going to be 12 to 15 Newtown officers who are going to be dealing with that, for the remainder of their careers, we imagine, from what we've been told by professionals who deal with PTSD."

PTSD, once associated primarily with soldiers, is now a well-recognized syndrome in police officers as well. Years ago, before much was known about PTSD (not a recognized diagnosis until 1980), noted crime author Joseph Wambaugh vividly described a police officer suffering PTSD symptoms in *The Onion Field*, his superb 1973 book, which was later made into a movie starring James Woods and Ted Danson.

During an uneventful patrol on a moonlit Southern California night in 1963, two Los Angeles policemen, Ian Campbell and Karl Hettinger, noticed a suspicious vehicle with two men in it. After pulling the car over, Campbell, the senior officer, approached and asked the driver to exit the car.

Events then took a horrific turn. Campbell was unaware the driver, Gregory Powell, a career criminal, had a concealed gun under the driver's seat. As Powell exited the car, he maneuvered the gun with his foot, emerged holding the weapon, and quickly subdued the unsuspecting Campbell. Powell, his gun in Campbell's back, then ordered Hettinger to surrender his service revolver. At first Hettinger refused, but with his partner's life at stake, he reluctantly gave up his gun.

Powell and his accomplice then kidnapped the two disarmed officers and drove them to a secluded rural road in an onion field about one hundred miles away. They shot and killed Campbell, but just as they were about to kill Hettinger, a cloud obscured the moonlight, and Hettinger escaped in the darkness and confusion.

The two criminals were soon captured and convicted, and received long prison sentences. Campbell, married and a father of two young daughters, had a police burial with full honors, including a team of bagpipers playing "Amazing Grace," a Los Angeles Police Department tradition since his death.

Wambaugh, a fellow L.A. police officer, decided to write *The Onion Field* because of what happened to the surviving officer, Karl Hettinger. After the incident, the LAPD was only vaguely aware of the overwhelming guilt Hettinger was experiencing. Police brass sent him to police roll calls across Los Angeles and ordered him to describe the events of that evening, how he surrendered his weapon, and the devastating consequences. Being forced to recount the details over and over simply reinforced his anguish and the feeling that he was somehow responsible for Campbell's death.

Depressed and finding it difficult to function, Hettinger was transferred to a less stressful job as a driver for the police chief, but he soon began shoplifting openly in front of people. He stole trivial items he did not need, and his behavior became so brazen he was forced to resign from the police force. He became a gardener in Los Angeles, and before dying in 1994, he relocated to Bakersfield, close to the onion field murder site, an intriguing postscript.

Hettinger's tragic circumstance inspired policeman-turned-author Wambaugh, who was quoted as saying,

> There wasn't anything said in those days about post-traumatic stress syndrome, let alone as it affects police officers. Nobody talked about that, but I was thinking about it, there has got to be a story here. This honest cop is running around stealing everything he can get his hands on. Sounds to me like guilt crying out for punishment. I thought if I ever become a writer, I'd sure like to look into this. . . . Sending that guy to roll calls and making him describe how he "screwed up" that night by surrendering his weapon. That kind of thing was probably more destructive to his psyche than the killing in the onion field. And what nearly destroyed him was the way that he was treated by the police department, but with no ill will and no malice. They didn't know what they were doing to the guy, it was just ignorance.

In 2013 on the fiftieth anniversary of the onion field murder, a sign was dedicated near the intersection of the traffic stop in memory of Ian Campbell. The LAPD has revised their procedures, advising officers never to surrender their weapons. Some closure was reached after Gregory Powell died in prison in 2012. (His accomplice died years ago.)

Shakespeare cautioned us to remember that what's past is prologue. Today we understand PTSD far better, but the pall it casts never completely disappears. Now that lingering pall is thousands of miles away from Los Angeles in distant Newtown.

17

NOTORIOUS PATIENTS: THE BOSTON MARATHON BOMBER

The evil that men do lives after them;
the good is oft interrèd with their bones.

—WILLIAM SHAKESPEARE, *JULIUS CAESAR*

WHEN DZHOKHAR TSARNAEV, the Boston Marathon bomber, was brought bleeding and wounded into the emergency room at Boston's Beth Israel Deaconess Medical Center, the staff faced a distressing predicament. How would the nurses and physicians take care of an especially notorious patient, one whose values are inimical to society?

As one trauma nurse who cared for Tsarnaev during his first night in the hospital explained it to the *Boston Globe*, "I am compassionate, that's what we do. But should I be? The rest of the world hates him right now. The emotions are like one big salad, all tossed around."

Everyone who treated Tsarnaev will struggle with those emotions for a long time. Every health professional in the emergency room and intensive care unit learns to treat felons, murderers, and rapists. Working in those particular hospital areas generally does not permit staff the luxury of refusing to treat a patient, no matter how odious that person may be. When something like the Boston Marathon bombing happens, the usual approach is to view the offender as simply another patient, just part of the hospital routine.

While that may be an adequate defense mechanism when caregivers treat most criminals, treating particularly heinous suspects, in this case an alleged terrorist, can be more complicated. For these kinds of patients, many in the public ask caregivers, "How can you take care of that person? Why do you do it?" The short but incomplete answer is it is part of the code nurses and physicians live by. But in reality, caring for patients like Tsarnaev compels even the most hardened nurse or physician to undergo some uncomfortable introspection. As that Boston trauma nurse added, "You see a hurt 19-year-old and you can't help but feel sorry for him," yet she said she "would not be upset if he got the death penalty. There is no way to reconcile the two different feelings."

I have heard military physicians who cared for enemy prisoners of war express similar sentiments. That internal conflict can be difficult to reconcile when you work in the hospital, especially when you are tasked with saving the life or relieving the suffering of someone who has maliciously taken innocent lives or caused others to suffer. Moreover, the constraints of confidentiality often prohibit caregivers from discussing details outside the hospital about the care they give to a high-profile patient. Not being able to share your feelings about treating the subject of national or international headlines can be stressful.

One final thing about caring for patients like Tsarnaev: there is something about them that will always be etched in your memory. Doctors and nurses generally forget most of the patients they treat in the course of their professional careers. But not in cases like this. No doctor or nurse at Beth Israel is likely to forget Tsarnaev. Each may have a different memory of some specific detail about treating him, but those details will remain with the workers for the rest of their lives. A physician I knew once cared for a notorious convicted murderer who tortured his victims before killing them. Years later, my colleague was able to describe in vivid detail the fear this murderer had of needles; the irony of a sadistic killer who could not bear the smallest needle for a tetanus shot or to have his blood drawn.

For me it was the faces. Many years ago, I briefly treated three people convicted of particularly gruesome crimes—one was an infamous serial killer, another was a mass murderer, and the third a mother who killed her child. All three, now dead for many years, made national headlines. Even today, decades later, I remember how each would stare at me menacingly when I came near them. It was chilling.

Things like that stay with you. There is something about certain patients you can never forget, and the Boston caregivers may unfortunately learn that about Dzhokhar Tsarnaev.

18

BORN TO RAISE HELL

The Lord saw that the wickedness of man was great in the earth,
and that every intention of the thoughts of his heart
was only evil continually.

—GENESIS 6:5

HAD MY FIRST REAL EXPERIENCE with evil in the world fifty years ago when I was twelve. In the summer of 1966, some friends and I went to the local news agency, where we were offered one dollar a day to wrap copies of the afternoon *Chicago Daily News*, ride in an old Pontiac with a chain-smoking delivery guy, and throw papers on the lawns of a new suburban subdivision. Good pay, unless you pitched a paper on the roof of a house. You got one mulligan—the second time you worked for free.

As I wrapped papers on my first week, the prominent front-page head-line was about eight student nurses stabbed and strangled to death by an unknown assailant in a Chicago townhouse. In 1966 mass murder on that scale was incomprehensible. Even by the grim calculus of Chicago homicide, Al Capone's gunmen killed only seven hoodlums in the notorious 1929

St. Valentine's Day Massacre. This new crime received instant worldwide attention ("went viral" in today's vernacular), and Chicagoans and suburbanites, myself included, were gripped by fear of a nameless psychopathic killer on the loose.

As a youngster, I, like so many others, was introduced to violent death by the 1963 John F. Kennedy assassination. The next year, three civil rights workers were brutally slain in Mississippi. But I was too young to comprehend the enormity of those events.

Now I was older, and this was local. Most unsettling was that front page I wrapped over and over again; it carried a police artist's sketch of the killer, created through details provided by the plucky young nurse who rolled under a bed and remained there all night, lying near the bodies of her lifeless friends.

That day, unnerved, I threw papers on the roofs of my first two houses. I didn't get paid, and it appeared I wasn't long for the job. The sketch was indelibly etched in my mind—a man with a crew cut; a thin, tapering face devoid of emotion; and cold, menacing eyes. That such a predator lurked somewhere chilled me to my bones. The surviving nurse provided another detail in her description of the killer—a BORN TO RAISE HELL tattoo on his arm (rendering him even more terrifying). This too was on the front page, and three days later, a young surgeon at Cook County Hospital was summoned to the new trauma unit to examine an alcoholic drifter who had attempted to commit suicide by slashing his wrists. After scrubbing blood from the drifter's arm, the doctor recognized the tattoo and checked the sketch in a newspaper. The mass murderer Richard Speck was captured. The police sketch turned out to be uncannily accurate except for the hair—not a crew cut, simply slicked back, an understandable mistake.

I soon squared myself with the news agency and kept newspapers off the roofs. But there were more headlines coming: violence and death would become routine in 1966. Two weeks later, Charles Whitman, an ex-marine and University of Texas student, killed his wife and her mother, then climbed to the top of the university clock tower with a high-powered rifle and killed fourteen more people. Within days of the Speck and Whitman murders, Rev. Martin Luther King Jr. came to Chicago to lead marchers protesting housing segregation. In an all-white neighborhood, the marchers were taunted by a group of local thugs, one of whom carried a sign reading KING WOULD LOOK GOOD WITH A KNIFE IN HIS BACK. Suddenly, on that sultry August afternoon, the marchers were showered with rocks and bottles. King was felled by a brick that struck him in the head.

Later that summer, less than ten miles from my home, Valerie Percy, the twenty-one-year-old daughter of then Senate candidate Charles Percy, was killed by a nocturnal intruder who entered the family's home in Kenilworth through a glass door just like one my family had. The killer was never caught, and for months I imagined him invading our house the same way.

The backdrop to all this was the Vietnam War. In 1966 more than six thousand American soldiers died in Vietnam (more than in the entire Iraq War), five times as many as in 1965. The Vietnam War death rate for Americans rose faster in that year than in any other year of the war.

Fast-forward twenty-five years. As the head of the intensive care unit at Cook County Hospital, I was called to see a high-profile prisoner having chest pain who was in town for some legal hearing. It was Richard Speck. Instantly, my mind raced back to that police sketch in the *Daily News*. Like a computer re-creation of someone aging, he resembled the sketch—but only barely. His pockmarked face was much fleshier and had taken on female characteristics. He had been taking female hormones, grown breasts, and gained weight. But the sinister visage was unchanged. Before I sent him to the cardiac unit, he made some cheap, sarcastic remark that bespoke pure evil. I sensed no remorse in his taunting smile. That was the only time I ever saw Speck.

Another twenty-five years have passed, but to this day that name reawakens that chill in my spine and the frisson of fear I felt when I was twelve.

19

WHO WAS NANCY REAGAN'S FATHER?

My name is Ozymandias, King of Kings;
Look on my Works, ye Mighty, and despair!
Nothing beside remains.

—PERCY BYSSHE SHELLEY, "OZYMANDIAS"

THE OBITUARIES of Nancy Reagan concentrated on her devotion to the most important person in her life—her husband, President Ronald Reagan. Less attention was focused on her stepfather, Dr. Loyal Davis, unquestionably the second-most important person in her life and possibly in President Reagan's as well.

Davis, one of the preeminent neurosurgeons in Chicago in the mid-century, ruled the operating room at Passavant Memorial Hospital (now part of Northwestern Memorial Hospital) with an iron fist for more than thirty years. He could charitably be described as a larger-than-life character.

I encountered the legend of Loyal Davis indirectly in 1976, long after he had retired to Arizona. I was a senior in medical school taking my oral final exam in surgery, which was administered by another Northwestern surgery professor. The professor questioned me about anatomy and surgical technique, and I flailed for answers. An honors designation was out of the question; I prayed for a passing grade so I would not have to repeat six weeks of surgery. Then came his last question, which was not about anatomy or technique: "Who is Loyal Davis?"

The name sounded vaguely familiar, but I had no clue. Bluffing was impossible. With visions of another surgical rotation in my future, I gulped and said tremulously, "I don't know."

The sword of Damocles hung precariously over my head. Suddenly he shocked me and bellowed, "That's the right answer! That SOB thought everyone would remember him forever. I just love to hear students say they don't know who he is." It turned out the professor was trained by Davis, and every student was asked about Davis as part of his or her orals.

"All right, you passed—barely. Now get out of here." With a wry smile, the prof sent me on my way.

After that, I wanted to find out about Davis. He was one of the country's most distinguished surgeons, but by most accounts, he was not a nice man to work with or for. Imperious and a martinet both inside and outside the operating room, he was liked by some residents and students, hated by others, but feared by all. A summons to his office was an encounter to be dreaded.

Politically, Davis was a staunch conservative who detested socialized medicine and any other form of government intervention in medicine. He was quite outspoken, with hidebound views on issues medical and nonmedical. Although personally aloof, Davis took a liking to his new son-in-law when Nancy married Ronald Reagan in 1952. The father-in-law enjoyed sharing his political views with the actor, and many sources credit Davis with being among the most important people in the transformation of

Ronald Reagan from a liberal Democrat in the 1940s into the conservative Republican he became in the 1950s and for the rest of his life.

Two years after my exam, my roommate had the same surgical professor for his orals. Before his exam, I told him what the final question would be. My roommate wanted to know who Loyal Davis was so he could correctly answer the surgery professor. I told him but said, "If you trust me, you'll say you don't know." Sure enough, my roommate was asked the trick question and, demonstrating his trust in me, said he didn't know. I think he got an honors designation.

The epilogue to this story came a couple of years later, when Reagan was elected president and Loyal Davis recommended his partner, Dr. Daniel Ruge, to be Reagan's White House physician. Ruge accepted and handled the position masterfully. He especially distinguished himself in coordinating Reagan's care after the president's 1981 assassination attempt, when his life was truly in jeopardy.

Loyal Davis has been dead for more than thirty years. I'm sure most current medical students don't know the name, but I will not forget him. My old surgery professor would probably fail me today.

20

ELEMENTARY, MY DEAR WATSON

At lunch Francis (Crick) winged into The Eagle to tell everyone
within hearing distance that we had found the secret of life.

—JAMES WATSON

WHEN THE HISTORY of medicine in the late twentieth century
and early twenty-first century is written, one of the key figures
and greatest contributors will be a native Chicagoan who was not even
a physician. That man, James Watson, earned his place in the annals of
medicine as a molecular biologist and scientific visionary. In 1953 Watson,
along with Francis Crick and two less heralded scientists, Rosalind Franklin
and Maurice Wilkins, discovered the DNA double helix, a discovery that
provided the avenue for the current genetics revolution in medicine. (Some
have opined that Dr. Franklin should have shared the 1962 Nobel Prize in
Physiology or Medicine with Watson, Crick, and Wilkins, but the award
is limited to three people. In addition, she died four years before the prize
was awarded, and the honor is limited to living recipients.)

Their work was the starting point for the worldwide effort to sequence the human genome, the holy grail of man's unique genetic heritage. Translation of the human genome will change the practice of medicine more than the discovery of the microscope, anesthesia, or antibiotics. Physicians will eventually be able to practice medicine by tailoring care for each individual according to their genetic profile, something past generations of physicians could not have imagined.

More than a half century after his momentous discovery, Watson was involved in another step in the genetics revolution when he was presented with a custom-made DVD, which took two months and $2 million to produce. The DVD contained virtually his entire personal genome sequence, and even at that cost was truly a bargain because it was produced with new technology that afforded the cheapest, quickest complete human gene sequencing to date. By comparison the government's Human Genome Project's first reference genome, released in 2003, took over a decade and cost $3 billion to complete. Current advances in DNA testing and computer chip development will soon bring the cost of human genome identification down to a fraction of the cost of Watson's and will make the sequencing available in a matter of days.

Meanwhile, simple genetic tests, identifying small fractions of the entire genome, are becoming available for use in the physician's office. These tests have the theoretical ability to predict specifically which patients are likely to respond to different medications and what doses are most effective.

Genetics may change the practice of many specialties. Researchers have identified genes associated with higher risks of developing breast and ovarian cancer, as well as malignancies of the gastrointestinal tract. Based on genetic profiles, oncologists are creating strategies for early diagnosis and treatment of these tumors. Reproductive medicine and in vitro fertilization will benefit from improvements in genetic profiling. On the other end of life, researchers will soon understand more about the genetic mutations involved in the aging process and Alzheimer's disease.

One of medicine's great twentieth-century clinicians, William Bean, once wrote, "The one mark of maturity, especially in a physician, and perhaps it is even rarer in a scientist, is the capacity to deal with uncertainty." Though he knew nothing of the human genome, Bean understood that uncertainty was an inevitable part of medical practice. There would always be things that would remain unknown to medical science. If he were alive today, he'd tip his hat to James Watson, who, though he never cared for a single patient, was responsible for eliminating a bit of the uncertainty of medical practice through the discovery of the double helix and his work with the human genome.

21

THE SACRIFICE OF OUR VALIANT MEN AND WOMEN

The surgery of wounds arising in military service concerns the extraction of missiles. In city practice experience of these is but little, for very rarely even in a whole lifetime are there civil or military combats.

— HIPPOCRATES

THIS QUOTE BY HIPPOCRATES from the fifth century BC (often para-phrased and simplified as the more familiar "War is the only proper school of the surgeon") is evidence that since antiquity war has been a primary impetus for medical progress and specifically trauma care. The ancient Romans developed sophisticated field stations behind battle lines to treat wounded foot soldiers. To control hemorrhage, Roman surgeons refined the art of the tourniquet and practiced amputation to prevent the spread of gangrene.

In the Middle Ages, European surgeons routinely perfected their craft at so-called schools for surgery—the battlefield—where gunpowder caused injuries unknown outside combat. French surgeons, notably Ambrose Paré, employed innovative modes of therapy for war wounds. Paré used ligatures to tie off blood vessels after amputation and abjured the use of boiling oil to cauterize wounds. However, success was limited as a consequence of the notoriously poor hygiene on the battlefield.

During the Crimean War in the 1850s, the practice of nursing was revolutionized and dignified by the legendary Florence Nightingale. A decade later American nurses gained similar status and esteem during the Civil War, the first war in which triage of patients from the field was implemented on a large scale. In the Franco-Prussian and Boer Wars of the late nineteenth century, doctors discovered the value of antiseptic technique in penetrating gunshot wounds.

From a medical standpoint, the carnage of World War I produced advances in orthopedics, neurosurgery, and psychiatry, as well as measures to prevent the spread of infectious disease on the battlefield, including advanced wound antisepsis, tetanus antitoxin, and typhoid vaccination. Ironically, despite the lives saved by these interventions, the close quarters of trench warfare and military training and the ensuing demobilization at the end of the war gave rise to the influenza pandemic claiming more than fifty million victims worldwide—the deadliest epidemic in the history of mankind.

After blood typing was discovered in 1901 by Austrian physician Karl Landsteiner, direct blood transfusion from patient to patient became feasible but was limited throughout World War I because blood could not be stored for prolonged periods. The work of Bernard Fantus at Cook County Hospital led to the ability to preserve blood for ten days, an astounding advance. In 1937 Fantus established a "Blood Preservation Laboratory," later renamed the Cook County Blood Bank, the world's first blood bank for prolonged blood storage. Stored blood was used for transfusion during the Spanish Civil War and on a much greater scale in World War II.

Penicillin, discovered in 1928, was first used extensively in World War II. The effect was close to miraculous, both on wound infections and for bacterial pneumonia. Infected battle wounds had been the scourge of every previous war, and now penicillin saved countless soldiers. In addition the mortality rate from pneumonia, 18 percent in World War I, dropped to under 1 percent in World War II. From January to May 1942, four hundred million units of pure penicillin were manufactured. By the end of the war, American pharmaceutical companies were producing 650 billion units a month.

Combat surgeons became essential battlefield personnel in World War II, and that "greatest generation" of military physicians trained several future generations of surgeons. The training of these physicians played a large role in the subsequent development of trauma units in the United States. Many of these combat surgeons also served in the Korean War, where helicopters were first employed extensively to transport soldiers and the mobile army surgical hospital (MASH) unit was developed (think Elliot Gould, Donald Sutherland, and Sally Kellerman or, if you are a little younger, Alan Alda, Wayne Rogers, and Loretta Swit). The MASH units were designed to bring experienced surgeons closer to the front lines to operate on wounded soldiers more quickly. Along with improvements in the treatment of shock and hemorrhage, these units were demonstrably effective in reducing the mortality of wounded soldiers.

These innovations, along with extensive research on resuscitation in hemorrhagic shock during the Vietnam War, led to a dramatic fall in battlefield mortality. In World War II, 30 percent of all Americans seriously injured in combat died. In Vietnam, despite more lethal weapons, 15 to 25 percent of all serious wounds proved fatal.

The twenty-first-century wars in Iraq and Afghanistan accelerated the pace of medical miracles and changed the approach to battlefield medicine. Formerly, the guiding philosophy of military surgery was definitive wound repair as quickly as possible. Now more lives can be saved by emphasizing rapid control of bleeding in the field, on-site resuscitation, and after stabilization, transport of patients for definitive surgery to larger support hospitals in-country or in the case of more complex injuries, transfer back to the United States.

On the battlefield, small, mobile medical teams have been equipped with sophisticated equipment and drugs undreamed of in previous wars, including chemically treated bandages that stop bleeding, genetically engineered drugs to promote clotting, and portable diagnostic ultrasound equipment. In the second Gulf War, once a severely injured patient was stabilized, the average transport time to a US facility from a Middle Eastern battlefield was four days compared to forty-five days from Vietnam back to the United States in the 1960s.

These advances, along with the refinement of Kevlar body armor and helmets, kept the harrowing figures of nearly seven thousand American deaths in Iraq and Afghanistan from being much higher. The mortality rate for wounded soldiers was somewhere between 8 and 12 percent. Given equivalent injuries, today's soldier is 50 percent less likely to die than his Vietnam counterpart fifty years ago.

The Vietnam-era adage "war is unhealthy for children and other living things" remains truer today than ever, but it is reassuring to realize that the knowledge gained and the techniques perfected in battlefield care are ultimately applied to civilian medicine and especially to today's trauma units. While far preferable to the alternative of "toe tags and body bags," lifesaving medical advances result in greater numbers of unfortunate soldiers surviving with severe brain injuries, paralyzing spinal cord damage, or overwhelming psychological trauma. These harrowing sequelae of combat must be addressed, not only by the medical community but also by society at large. And ultimately, no matter what the political outcome of war, all Americans benefit from the sacrifice of our valiant men and women.

III

HOSPITALS AND HOSPITAL
PRACTICES: *THE TWILIGHT ZONE*

22

HOSPITALS: SCARY PLACES EVEN FOR DOCTORS

Even top caliber hospitals cannot escape medical mistakes that sometimes result in irreparable damage to patients.

—Senator Carl Levin

THE MAN HAD BEEN VOMITING, was incoherent, and reeked of alcohol. Believing it to be a routine "drunk call," the ambulance drivers took their time transporting him to the emergency room. Once at the hospital, he lay on a stretcher for some time, unattended, because the medical staff too believed he was just one more guy who'd had one too many. It happens almost every night in the emergency room to some poor John Doe. Except that the man wasn't drunk. He had been beaten and robbed on his way home from dinner. His medical evaluation was delayed for several critical hours before the staff realized their error, and he died two days later as a result of blunt trauma to the head, neck, and torso.

Cases like that don't happen often, but one of the more common emergency room errors is mistaking a medically ill patient for one who is merely drunk. Most patients who smell of alcohol or have a high blood alcohol content are merely intoxicated and will be fine in several hours as the alcohol is metabolized. But in a small number of those patients, alcohol masks other conditions—trauma, infections, diabetic coma—that must be treated immediately. A delay of several hours is often the difference between life and death.

One of the startling things about this case was this John Doe victim turned out to be a reporter for the *New York Times*. Several years before that, another highly publicized medical error occurred when the medical reporter for the *Boston Globe* died after receiving the wrong dose of chemotherapy. Errors or near errors have occurred involving family members of some of the most well-known physicians in the country, including the wives of Donald Berwick, the president of the Institute of Healthcare Improvement, and Albert Wu, one of the country's leading internists from Johns Hopkins. If it can happen to these people, it can happen to anybody. So far every doctor I have talked to has shuddered and agreed with that basic premise.

Physicians are familiar with the errors, both trivial and serious, endemic to hospitals. Yet even with their medical expertise, hospital connections, and familiarity with the inner workings of the system, physicians are often powerless to prevent hospital danger and indignity. Wrong medications dispensed, miscommunications at shift changes, and tests continually rescheduled are all common screwups. In addition hospital care is increasingly dictated by specialists. Patients may benefit from doctors who are better informed, but a lack of coordinated effort between specialists sometimes results in confusing and contradictory treatment plans.

The people running hospitals have only now begun to remedy these problems. Today hospital marketing arms have photogenic doctors striding confidently around the "campus" (the current pretentious term) describing the wonderful things going on all around them. On its best days, that's what the hospital is like: effective care, compassion, and the occasional miracle. When you're sick, you hope that's what you get. Of course when you go to Wrigley Field (unless you're a White Sox fan), you hope the Cubs play errorless ball, hit home runs, and pitch shutouts. But ultimately at the hospital and the ballpark, hope and reality don't always jibe. Hospitals can be wonderful places, but they can also be bastions of miscommunication, inefficiency, indifference, and bureaucracy that would make a Third World post office look impressive.

There are some things a smart patient can do:

Bring someone who can stay with you. The hospital can be a lonely and frightening place. A trusted family member or friend can be invaluable, especially on weekends and holidays.

Ask questions. Not in a way that questions authority (the staff is human, they don't like that) but in a way that shows interest and concern with your health. Contrary to popular opinion, most doctors and nurses like it when patients ask questions. It gives them a chance to involve you in your care, bond with you, and show off their knowledge a little bit (the staff is human, they do like that).

Also, a box of candy never hurts. Make it two, one for the doctors and one for the nurses.

In 2002 the Harvard School of Public Health reported over one-third of the doctors surveyed reported errors in either their own care or that of family members. The hospital can be as oblivious to the patient concerns of connected reporters or informed physicians as it is to everyone else. It recalls a joke comedian Richard Belzer once told: "When I hear Mick Jagger sing he can't get no satisfaction, I think if that's true, what chance does a poor guy like me have?"

23

ER OVERLOAD

People have access to health care in America.
After all, you just go to an emergency room.

—George W. Bush

THE SHOCKING RECORDING of the 911 call suggested the dispatcher had no idea what to do when she received a call from the boyfriend of Edith Isabel Rodriguez. As he pleaded with the dispatcher to send paramedics to her aid, Rodriguez lay on the floor, in pain, throwing up blood. The dispatcher was flummoxed, though, because the policy of "take the patient to the closest hospital" didn't apply. Rodriguez was already in the emergency room lobby of Los Angeles' inner-city Martin Luther King Jr.–Harbor Hospital.

Shortly after another bystander made a second futile 911 call imploring paramedics to take Rodriguez to another hospital, she died of a perforated bowel. A security videotape was said to show her writhing on the hospital floor unattended for forty-five minutes. At one point the tape reportedly showed a janitor going about his business mopping the floor around her. A number of staff were merely reprimanded over the incident.

Her death became the center of a controversy in Los Angeles, typifying the bureaucratic indifference of a public hospital that treats primarily indigent and minority patients. This case involving King-Harbor prompted federal inspection of the medical center even as politicians and physicians pointed fingers at each other. Ultimately, in large part because of the Rodriguez case, the hospital closed and reopened as a smaller facility nearly a decade later.

Edith Rodriguez's death struck a special nerve throughout Southern California, where even the wealthy often endure interminable waits in the emergency room. For the poor, the situation is worse because the emergency room is often the only place they can go to see a doctor. In Rodriguez's case, she died with nurses and doctors literally in the next room. The Rodriguez case exemplifies our public health care system at its worst. Similar tragedies have occurred at public hospitals in other cities, but this problem is not confined to the public sector: in 1998, a boy bled to death after being shot right outside the emergency room of one of Chicago's North Side private hospitals.

The media that profess shock at public hospital ineptitude often fail to mention the complicity of bureaucrats, politicians, and the private hospital system, all of which contribute to the big picture. After the controversy over the Rodriguez case, Los Angeles was the scene of another scandal when certain private hospitals were discovered to have arranged for ambulances to discharge indigent and disabled patients to a skid row area.

Unfortunately, there are no simple solutions to tragedies such as that of Edith Isabel Rodriguez. Deaths such as hers are usually the result of a combination of administrative incompetence, medical and nursing negligence, bureaucratic indifference, and emergency room overcrowding. The last is a particularly vexing problem across the country. Emergency room overcrowding is usually a result of a dysfunctional primary care system, a problem not unique to Los Angeles. Too many people forced to visit the emergency room for primary care renders the emergency room not only inconvenient but also occasionally dangerous. It may be worse in the public sector, but patients often have to wait a long time in fancy private emergency rooms too.

Without a fundamental restructuring of primary care, emergency rooms will continue to serve as the clinic of last resort, a situation that benefits no one. It is ironic that for decades the American public hospital system represented the best and worst of our society. The best because it took care of those the system otherwise ignored. The worst because of the incompetence and indifference that cost the lives of Edith Isabel Rodriguez and so many others like her.

24

PROTECT PATIENTS' MEDICAL RECORDS FROM PRYING EYES

Progress is man's ability to complicate simplicity.

—THOR HEYERDAHL

I N TODAY'S MODERN WORLD, certain developments demand a wellspring of public outrage. A case in point should be the results of a study published in *JAMA: The Journal of the American Medical Association* that went virtually unnoticed. The study found that between 2009 and 2013, more than twenty-nine million medical records were hacked, stolen, or otherwise compromised. Most of these were criminal breaches, with five states—California, Florida, Illinois, New York, and Texas—accounting for 34 percent of all breaches.

The study's lead author, Dr. Vincent Liu, estimated the actual number was likely even larger. He believes the trend of medical record theft will continue unabated in the future. "Our study demonstrates that data breaches have been and will continue to be a persistent threat to patients, clinicians and health care systems," Liu said.

In the last twenty years, the electronic medical record has been promoted by the government and health care industry as a way to improve care, save money, and, not surprisingly, process payment. As the *JAMA* study indicated, an unforeseen consequence of the transition from paper to computerized records means that even with passwords, firewalls, and encryption software, your medical file can be accessed anywhere in the world. This means not just your diagnoses, test results, and insurance information but your home address, social security number, employment data, genetic profile, and other confidential personal information.

Since the time of Hippocrates, about twenty-five hundred years ago, medical confidentiality has been the cornerstone ensuring patients could communicate freely with their caregivers. Confidentiality guaranteed that the interests of patients and caregivers were aligned, so patients could receive care and doctors could render it without fear of divulging information publicly.

For decades your medical records were reasonably secure. Hospitals, clinics, and doctors maintained the traditional presumption of confidentiality; records were usually kept as paper charts stored in an office or hospital basement. Insurance company billing required only a few pages, not a complete set of medical records. It was certainly possible for an unauthorized person to examine or steal a patient's chart, but these were isolated occurrences. Those truly intent on mischief could do so only by surreptitiously removing a record and copying it. Even then, only a limited number of copies could be generated. The worst problems occurred due to the occasional improper disposal of paper medical records; in such incidents, at most several hundred records might be breached. Nothing on the scale of millions of records being compromised was conceivable, let alone possible.

Enter the electronic medical record. Its introduction has provided undeniable advantages to medical care, including making health records immediately accessible to providers, avoiding duplicated testing, allowing doctors at distant centers to see information instantaneously, and providing patients the ability to transfer their records to other providers easily. (These advantages unfortunately have not always included giving patients copies of their medical records without charging the patient exorbitant fees.) Yet as the medical community is painfully finding out, the electronic medical record has not been an unalloyed benefit.

Entering information into a computer while doing a medical interview has depersonalized the patient encounter to the detriment of the patient and the profession. It takes an exorbitant amount of the professional's time. In addition reams of extraneous and duplicated information mean a simple hospital stay of several days now results in a virtually unreadable thousand-page chart printout.

But the most serious unintended problem of the computerized record has been the sacrifice of patient privacy and security of personal health information. Records have been breached on levels undreamed of only several years ago. With a little expertise, almost any computerized patient chart can be copied and distributed over the Internet to anyone in seconds. And even a single stolen laptop can contain thousands of patient files. It would be hard to conceive of a more inviting platform to identity theft.

Recently hackers targeted the health insurance giant Anthem and made the personal information of nearly eighty million Americans vulnerable, only one example of the massive security problem. An article in the blog *Fast Company* claims that on the dark web, hacked medical records go for four times the price of stolen social security numbers and twenty times the price of stolen credit cards.

There is no ready solution to this problem. Experts can devise new encryption systems to thwart hackers, but eventually the malefactors will beat any system. At the same time, the harder it is to access records, the more it bollixes up medical care, because consultants, nurses, and parapro-fessionals must be able to access patient information. Our medical records are now perpetually vulnerable; it's simply a question of how much incon-venience we are willing to tolerate to frustrate hackers temporarily.

By themselves, patients have little recourse. Both the medical and legal communities, including the American Medical Association and the American Civil Liberties Union, must take a much stronger stand on the behalf of patients and make the safety of personal health information a higher priority. More state and federal legislation is necessary, because there are major holes in the way current laws are written. As experts have pointed out, digital information companies such as Apple, Google, and Facebook, with the potential to access patients' medical information, are not covered by most health care regulations. Further, computer outlaws, including offshore hackers, are hardly deterred by American law.

Welcome to the brave new world of health care. Computerized medical records have given your health care providers better access to your medical information than ever before, even while your medical history will never again be as secure as that of your grandparents. Most people in health care consider this progress. But as George Orwell once observed, progress is invariably disappointing.

25

RETRACING YOUR FOOTSTEPS

Do not follow where the path may lead.

—Ralph Waldo Emerson

SOMETIMES WHEN YOU'RE HIKING, if you inadvertently stray too far into the forest, the best thing to do is just admit that you took the wrong trail. Likewise, after three decades of experimenting, it should be time for the medical community to concede that the adoption of the electronic medical record (EMR) was a mistake and has been more detrimental than beneficial to patient care.

Unfortunately, in this case, what's done cannot be undone. It certainly seemed like a good idea in the early 1990s, at a time when patients began seeing many different doctors and frequenting many different hospitals, to develop a computerized system that would collect large amounts of information and make it available anywhere and anytime. When the government effectively mandated that all health care providers adopt EMRs, the plan was poorly conceived, with insufficient input by the professionals who would ultimately use digital records and without much forethought or actual evidence to support the benefit. This in the face of health care ombudsmen constantly criticizing medical practitioners for practicing without good evidence.

The thought was that medical records are similar to bank or other business records. They aren't, and it's much harder to develop workable digital systems. Different health care settings, specialties, and practitioners all require different types of records. A rural primary care clinic needs a different medical record than a university hospital ophthalmology department. This created a new multibillion-dollar nationwide industry for maintaining and updating medical records, so the toothpaste is out of the tube.

In fairness the new system has resulted in improvements in information retrieval and portability—at a huge cost. The government and the private sector spent billions of dollars and created a vast new bureaucracy to replace the paper medical record. Soon hospitals could not run without huge IT departments (the cost of which has become part of those egregious hospital bills).

What was the result of all this? Almost thirty years later, there is no single, universally accepted, user-friendly EMR system, and worse, no promise there will ever be one. The current systems usually cannot communicate with each other, and they all cost millions of dollars and require continual updating and maintenance (and once again, this becomes part of those hospital bills). Whether care is better is an unanswered question.

In addition the EMR was supposed to reduce paperwork, but when a paper copy of a chart is required for any reason today, it can result in thousands of pages of unreadable, superfluous information. Recently I saw a printout of a patient's hospitalization that was over eight thousand pages, probably ten times as many pages as her entire paper medical record since birth.

The most pernicious aspect of all this has been that in many cases, the EMR has become a wedge between patients and caregivers. I hear patients complain that their physician spends more time looking at the computer than looking at them. A recent study found doctors in training spend only 12 percent of their time in direct patient care compared with 40 percent of time spent in front of computers. At the same time, physicians complain more and more about the extra hours they spend in the hospital or clinic because documenting a patient encounter in the EMR takes more time than actually seeing the patient.

Without question, the EMR has certain advantages. Some advocates counter the pessimism over EMRs with stories of how the systems facilitate retrieval of patient labs, X-rays, and medications; how poor penmanship is no longer a problem; and how easy it is to access the latest medical literature. Yet those things could have been accomplished for a fraction of the expense without undermining the system that existed, by implementing computerized retrieval of clinical information in a more limited fashion.

And although no one would admit this, the primary value of the EMR currently resides not as an aid to patient care but in its reliability as an efficient record of things the hospital can charge for (charges that no one can explain anyway). Thus hospitals collecting medical payments have no incentive to change the system. Moreover, a whole generation of physicians, nurses, and health care personnel has grown up knowing nothing but the computer. (The other day on the hospital ward, I asked if anyone had a pencil and was met with strange looks all around.) It would seem hopelessly Luddite for a hospital or clinic to revert to the paper record, no matter its advantages.

Some experts insist that EMRs are still in their infancy and that eventually a single, workable system will be developed. If anything the problem is far more intractable than it was three decades ago. Future improvements in the EMR are likely to occur only at the margins of the technology and will likely be of more benefit to hospital collection than to patients.

There is little anyone can do about the state of affairs. One suggestion would be for patients to develop their own condensed personal medical record, especially for clinic visits. With help from their physicians, patients could carry a list of their conditions, medications, important lab tests, and a summary of their doctors' findings, updated after every clinic visit. It won't replace the EMR, but it might help caregivers who see patients.

Sadly, patients and their caregivers are destined to remain captives of the dysfunctional EMR. It is here to stay and will change the practice of medicine irrevocably. There is no going back: as any experienced hiker can tell you, once you go deep enough in the forest, you can't count on retracing your footsteps.

26

MEDICAL PROTOCOLS AND CHECKLIST MANIFESTOS

Our ideas must be as broad as Nature
if they are to interpret Nature.

—Sir Arthur Conan Doyle

IN HIS INFLUENTIAL BOOK *A Checklist Manifesto,* Dr. Atul Gawande describes how simple checklists can revolutionize medicine. The use of hospital checklists has already produced significant benefits, including fewer surgical mishaps and lower infection and hospital complication rates. Most checklists are simple and easy to understand, so outside review organizations have embraced them in the practice of medicine.

But improving medical care through checklists is not the sum and substance of practicing medicine, which requires accurate interpretation of patients' signs and symptoms, awareness and ability to assess treatment risks, and very often a sixth sense of when to act. Guidelines and protocols only describe these intangibles incompletely. As such, they are the GPS of medicine—they can make the journey easier, but it's best having a professional who knows the territory and terrain.

A current case in point is the plight of obstetricians/gynecologists, specifically regarding cesarean section and the timing of delivery. The American C-section rate has risen from 5 percent in 1970 to 32 percent today, a trend common to other parts of the world, with similarly high rates (and little financial incentive to perform C-sections) including South America, China, and Europe. When deciding to perform C-sections, physicians are responsible for the well-being of mother and baby; this means accounting for many complex factors. In the United States, the reasons for the C-section increase are primarily medical—greater use of drugs to induce labor, older and heavier mothers, higher rates of diabetes and other maternal diseases. An important nonmedical reason is the litigious environment, obstetrics being a fertile area (no pun intended) of medical malpractice claims; many physicians believe C-section reduces the risk of being sued.

Physicians also use fetal monitoring more often than in the past, which has created a concomitant trend toward delivery before the "ideal" delivery date of thirty-nine weeks. This is problematic because babies born before thirty-nine weeks have higher incidences of death and neurologic and pulmonary problems. Neonatal intensive care units nationwide are experiencing greater rates of admission, a tragic and extremely expensive problem. Understandably the government, the American College of Obstetricians and Gynecologists, and the Joint Commission on Accreditation of Hospitals (JCAH) have all put in motion efforts to decrease the rate of C-sections and eliminate nonmedically indicated deliveries before thirty-nine weeks. On its face this would seem to be a no-brainer. But it's not that simple.

Some ob-gyns worry that the drive to manage how and when delivery should occur could become a heavy-handed mandate tying doctors' hands. This concern deserves a hearing for several reasons. First, while earlier delivery and C-section result in greater neonatal morbidity and mortality only after the baby has been delivered, some literature suggests there are babies who would otherwise die in the womb but can be saved by delivery at thirty-seven or thirty-eight weeks. Hence the decision when to deliver becomes a delicate balance. Second, "nonmedical" indications can be vague; some diseases of mother and fetus are subtle. To diagnose correctly and intervene requires knowledge and judgment. Finally, doctors in the trenches are understandably reluctant to be judged harshly by hospital quality-indicator committees or the JCAH. Lawsuit or not, the physician attempting to do the right thing for the patient may find him- or herself abandoned if a delivery goes wrong.

The drive by outside organizations to improve obstetric and other medical care is commendable. But some doctors' fears of procrustean rules preventing them from practicing in the right manner are also real. No organization currently mandates a specific C-section rate or time for delivery, but it is not hard to see how "one size fits all" recommendations might eventually become a standard of care. Doctors deal with the uniqueness of each case, honing their ability and skill to recognize inevitable outliers. They don't want to see that ability hampered by a spate of rules and regulations.

In 1847 the man who ultimately became history's most famous obstetrician noticed that pregnant women in Vienna were six times more likely to die if delivered by physicians than if delivered by midwives. Decades before the cause of infections was known, Ignaz Semmelweis realized the deaths were due to "putrid material"—that is, bacteria doctors unknowingly transmitted to women. He believed the doctors, who did not wear gloves and worked in the autopsy lab before going to the delivery area, picked up this material in the lab. He felt strongly that virtually all the deaths could be prevented if the doctors simply washed their hands with household bleach before attending the women (presaging Gawande's checklists).

Influential idea, but stubborn European obstetricians refused to wash their hands, reviled Semmelweis, and tragically destroyed his medical career. Eventually his controversial recommendation was vindicated, saving countless women. Today, reputation restored, he is recognized as the pioneer of hand-washing and antisepsis, a medical giant with clinics and a university named for him.

Critics point to the story of Semmelweis and his detractors as proof of the medical establishment's long-standing arrogance and dogmatism. The indictment has some merit, but those who do point to this miss something else in the story—the hero who revolutionized medicine was not some bureaucratic organization but a brilliant, iconoclastic physician. In the new organizational world where shadow practitioners may dictate medical rules though protocols, might the next Semmelweis go forever undiscovered?

27

AN AMERICAN DISGRACE

Caring for veterans shouldn't be a partisan issue.
It should be an American one.
—GOVERNOR JENNIFER GRANHOLM

SURELY WE OWE OUR VETERANS better than the enduring travesty of what is happening at our veterans' hospitals. As part of the ongoing national scandal, the Department of Veterans Affairs' Office of Inspector General revealed that in 2014 and 2015 staff at Houston-area Veterans Affairs (VA) facilities improperly manipulated over two hundred wait times for Texas veterans looking to schedule medical appointments at VA clinics. By shifting the blame for cancellations from the staff to patients, VA employees made it appear waiting times for clinic visits were shorter than they really were. Veterans often waited an average of nearly three months for rescheduled appointments.

Even worse, this nationwide embarrassment is a recurring problem. In 2014 VA employees in Phoenix, Arizona, entered false dates into the

appointment system, so veterans waited far longer than the recorded waiting times—with some patients dying as a result. That scandal cost then VA
secretary Eric Shinseki his position and prompted a massive reform effort,
which obviously didn't make its way to Houston anytime soon. The federal
report states, "These issues have continued despite the Veterans Health
Administration having identified similar issues during a May and June
2014 system-wide review of access. . . . These conditions persisted because
of a lack of effective training and oversight. . . . Wait times did not reflect
the actual wait experienced by the veterans and the wait time remained
unreliable and understated."

And waiting times are only one problem among many. The appalling
rates of severe post-traumatic stress disorder and suicide among veterans
remain unacceptably high. Besides that, in the decade after 9/11, the Department of Veterans Affairs paid out $200 million to nearly one thousand
families in wrongful death cases.

The experience of former marine and Massachusetts representative Seth
Moulton (D) tells much about the system. It took Representative Moulton,
a veteran of four tours in Iraq, over a half hour at a Washington, DC, VA
hospital just to prove he was a veteran. When he sought care, he did not
have his VA card. Opting not to identify himself as a congressman but
simply as a veteran, he provided what should have been sufficient identification while observing other veterans who had been sitting in the waiting
room for hours.

He described to NPR what happened: "I checked in at the front desk,
and about 30 minutes later, they told me that they had no record of me.
They couldn't prove that I was a veteran. But they would consider taking
me as a humanitarian case. . . . [They had] more than enough things to put
into their computer system, supposedly the world-renowned VA computerized medical records system. . . . If that's the care they're giving to a United
States congressman, you can imagine what the average veteran is getting at
many of the VA facilities across the country." (The VA has since adopted
a new computer system.)

But the system apparently rewards failure; after officials covered up an outbreak of Legionnaires' disease at a Pittsburgh VA that left at least sixteen veterans ill and six dead, the VA regional director, Michael Moreland, received a nearly $63,000 bonus. Amid all this, VA secretary Robert McDonald didn't exactly inspire public confidence in 2016 when he compared VA care to a trip to Disneyland. He said of the long wait times that veterans must experience for clinic visits, "When you go to Disney, do they measure the number of hours you wait in line? Or what's important? What's important is, what's your satisfaction with the experience?" (In fact Disney does indeed track how long visitors wait in line for attractions at its theme parks—but that's beside the point.)

When the agency tried to walk back McDonald's obtuse remarks, it doubled down on the patient satisfaction meme: "We know that veterans are still waiting too long for care. In our effort to determine how we can better meet Veterans' needs, knowing that their satisfaction is our most important measure, we have heard them tell us that wait times alone are not the only indication of their experience with the VA."

To be clear—in any hospital patient satisfaction is one, but only one, measure of care. The most important measures are how patients' health and quality of life are being managed. Are acute diseases being diagnosed and treated correctly? Are chronic diseases being managed adequately? Is appropriate screening being performed? Is the quality of life being addressed in those with mental and physical disabilities? Those things should be the secretary's primary concern, as well as the primary concern of the thousands of VA employees.

Like Eric Shinseki, McDonald has since been replaced (which means the VA has had three directors in less than five years), and although McDonald's remarks seem to have come out of Fantasyland, where a loop of "It's a Small World" plays continuously, the VA health care system is not Disneyland. The comparison betrays disrespect for veterans and suggests it is unlikely the system will be corrected any time soon.

When Shinseki was sacked after the Phoenix VA travesty, President Obama said, "We're going to do right by our veterans across the board, as long as it takes. We're not going to stop working to make sure that they get the care, the benefits and the opportunities that they've earned and they deserve. I said we wouldn't tolerate misconduct, and we will not. I said that we have to do better, and we will."

But we haven't. And the whole thing is an American disgrace.

28

THE FUTURE OF HEALTH CARE: MUCH LIKE THE PRESENT, ONLY LONGER

Life can only be understood backwards;
but it must be lived forward.

—SØREN KIERKEGAARD

L IKE AN OLD CAR WITH TOO MANY MILES, American health care
sputters along in a chronic state of disrepair. Although we pay more
than $3 trillion annually, our health care system is broken, with no quick
fix in sight. And in fact, it may be irreparably broken because each new
solution instituted by payers and providers, whether effective or not, results
in new, more insoluble problems.

Consider an important example of an increasingly dysfunctional solution: the logic of insurance payment systems. In *The Health Care Blog*,
radiologist Saurabh Jha explains how incomprehensible the system is. His

experience with Medicare and private insurers is that they would refuse payment when he believed that a preauthorized test was wasteful or dangerous and he wanted to perform a simpler, safer test. Essentially, if he did less and billed for less than what the insurer agreed upon, they would not pay for anything, leaving the patient to pay the bill.

Likewise, if he did more than what was preauthorized because he felt it was clinically indicated or might spare the patient future tests, the insurer, fearing fraud, would refuse all payment. In addition offering billable services to Medicare patients without billing Medicare, as an effort at charity care, put him at risk of the fraud laws—the government might actually consider charity care given to Medicare or Medicaid patients as fraud.

Jha wrote,

> The reason insurers, and Medicare, would rather pay more, than less, for an exam, that is cut off their nose to spite their face, is that they don't trust physicians. They don't trust physicians because fifty years of health economics has yielded a spectacular insight—physicians, like crack dealers, are guilty of supplier-induced demand. This meme is now structurally embedded in payers. The information to discern between physicians inducing their demand and physicians curbing their demand is too costly to obtain. So third party payers have a blanket rule—you can neither upgrade nor downgrade an imaging study, and if you do you'll be paid nothing or will be done for fraud. . . . A costly game of chicken is being played between payers and providers. It's a game of reverse chicken actually, where both sides avoid staring at each other, and adapt to each other's pathologies.

Welcome to what happens when insurers, government or private, manage care: waste, inefficiency, and aggravation. Our current bizarre system is the result of trying to correct the previous unworkable system, in which providers managed their own care and their income depended on provision of services. This resulted in too many tests and procedures. Again, no foreseeable solution, no matter what political party is in power.

Is the answer a single-payer system to eliminate waste and inefficiency? That is a fool's errand; one need only observe the egregious abuses in our veterans' health care system.

The basic problem is that health care has three aims: access for everyone, lower costs, and better quality. (Other industries have a similar triad: "faster, cheaper, better.") Nowhere in the world has any system figured out how to provide all three. Moreover, when a system makes an effort to provide one, either or both of the other two may suffer.

Western Europe prides itself on broad access for its citizens along with low costs, but in every Western European country, health care costs are outstripping the gross domestic product (and all this of course is financed by significant taxation). Like the United States, their systems are requiring ever-greater spending. Moreover, other countries with single-payer systems do not perform better. Our health care system is undeniably more wasteful but at the same time more technologically advanced and innovative than any in the world. America provides a medical tourism industry for the wealthy and powerful of other countries.

The Affordable Care Act (ACA) was an attempt to broaden access for all Americans, and it did, although it did not provide complete coverage for everyone. In addition health care costs continued to rise faster than the rate of inflation (although not as quickly as before the ACA was enacted), and there was no improvement in overall mortality in the United States (admittedly an incomplete measure of quality). Besides this, not everyone who liked his or her doctor was able to keep them. Only the most sanguine observer would take the position that the ACA solved the access/cost/quality issue. Nor is it likely any replacement plan will work any better. It may well be that the access/cost/quality problem is unsolvable through any all-encompassing approach.

Perhaps there is another way for policy makers to approach the problem. They have been trying to solve American health care ills with a top-down broad-system approach. Have they been attempting too much? It might be more effective for the government to attack smaller problems—

pharmaceutical prices, care for the indigent, the opiate and obesity crises—incrementally on a case-by-case basis.

No matter what is done, there is little reason to believe that twenty years down the line health care will be in any different state than it is now. In the words of baseball player Dan Quisenberry, "I have seen the future—and it is much like the present, only longer."

29

THE DIGITAL INTRUSION INTO HEALTH CARE AND THE CREEPY LINE

And worse I may be yet: the worst is not
So long as we can say "This is the worst."

— WILLIAM SHAKESPEARE, *KING LEAR*

I N 2010 TOP Google executive Eric Schmidt told the *Atlantic*, "Google policy is to get right up to the creepy line and not cross it. . . . We know where you are. We know where you've been. We can more or less know what you're thinking about."

Whether it intended to or not, Google has now crossed the creepy line—with ominous implications for patients everywhere. It partnered in a British medical project involving more than one million patients that was effectively hidden from the public until recently. The project's lack of concern for privacy and informed consent was blatant exploitation of these

111

patients, and unless greater attention is paid to digital companies entering the health care universe, the public will be at significant risk in the future.

It began, as so many notorious medical experiments do, with ostensibly good intentions. In 2015 Royal Free NHS Foundation Trust, which operates a number of British hospitals, entered into a seemingly benign agreement with a Google subsidiary, DeepMind. In an effort to develop an app to monitor patients at risk of kidney disease, DeepMind was granted access to the health information of 1.6 million patients. The assumption was that this information would be limited to factors related to kidney disease, but there was no explicit mention in the agreement of the nature or amount of data to be collected. Within months, Google-contracted servers were amassing sensitive personal medical information with little relation to kidney disease, from emergency room treatments to details of personal drug abuse.

Until journalists prompted a government investigation, DeepMind accessed the personally identifiable medical records of a large number of patients—with no guarantee of confidentiality, formal research protocol, research approval, or individual consent.

Also, neither Royal Free nor Google chose to explain why DeepMind, with virtually no health care experience, was selected for this project. Apparently neither British regulators nor physicians asked any substantive questions.

Elizabeth Denham of the UK Information Commissioner's Office, the ombudsman for the country's medical data, released a statement regarding a probe of the secretive DeepMind deal: "Our investigation found a number of shortcomings in the way patient records were shared for this trial. Patients would not have reasonably expected their information to have been used in this way, and the Trust could and should have been far more transparent with patients as to what was happening." An admirable, albeit belated, first step by the organization that failed to anticipate the obvious dangers of an arrangement between one of Britain's largest health care providers and the world's dominant data mining/advertising corporation.

There is, of course, a larger issue at stake, one that Denham failed to address. Medical information is the last fragile redoubt of our rapidly eroding personal privacy. While professing good intentions, Google has an unstated but obvious conflict of interest in the data mining of large populations. Did Google have an ulterior motive in collecting the medical information of such a huge patient cohort? And more important, when monolithic digital companies like Google, Microsoft, Apple, Facebook, and Amazon, which already control much of our personal and professional activity, enter the health care industry as they inevitably will, who will protect patients' interests?

Once these companies introduce artificial intelligence and proprietary algorithms into medical care, will there be transparency? If not, what recourse will the public have? One author has likened Google to a one-way mirror—it knows much about us and is learning more every day, but we really know virtually nothing about it. The paramount concern of any medical research is to preserve the rights of patients and subjects, and this one-way mirror does little to ensure that.

After the UK Information Commissioner's investigation, DeepMind cofounder Mustafa Suleyman assured the public that new safeguards would be instituted and that the company's goal is to have a positive social impact. We expect him to say that, but the twentieth century was replete with notorious studies that were kept secret or justified on the basis of their supposed societal benefit. If the history of medical ethics has taught us anything, it is that patients do not exist to serve medical science and that they must never be deprived of the right to control their medical treatment, regardless of researchers' stated beneficence.

Big data is coming to medicine, and it would be remiss not to acknowledge the potential benefits of machine learning and artificial intelligence. But no matter how valuable the promise of these new approaches and how well intentioned the motives of those responsible, without transparency, safeguards, and continual oversight, the seeds of abuse and tragedy are never far away. And here in the United States, will HIPPA offer sufficient protection?

Be forewarned, the story of Royal Free and Google DeepMind is a clarion call. It is merely the introductory chapter in a new marriage of health care and digital companies that seek to collect and control medical information. One is reminded of the warning given to Charles Foster Kane in *Citizen Kane*: "You're going to need more than one lesson, and you are going to get more than one lesson."

IV

RESEARCH, ETHICS, DRUGS, AND MONEY

30

SHOULD YOU PUT YOUR TRUST IN MEDICAL RESEARCH?

The saddest aspect of life right now is that science gathers
knowledge faster than society gathers wisdom.

—ISAAC ASIMOV

A FRIEND OF MINE, a physician with thirty years of experience in
medical research who has published in the world's top medical journals, recently said to me, "I don't believe most of the studies published in
the medical literature anymore." His candid skepticism was because he
feels medical researchers are losing the trust of the public.

Trust is an essential ingredient of medical research, and the accelerating
erosion of trust in the biomedical literature that my friend noted is the result
of several factors: fraud, conflicts of interest, and inadequate scientific and
journalistic peer review. These malign influences have corrupted scientific
literature for generations, but their current manifestations are particularly
acute in medical research.

A notable instance of fraud came to the fore in 2015 when the prestigious journal *Science*, thought by many to be the top science journal in the world, retracted a prominent paper on gay marriage after the lead author lied about certain features of the study. This high-profile retraction was only more evidence that fraud has become depressingly common in the biomedical literature.

A review of more than two thousand articles retracted by major journals revealed that more than two-thirds were retracted because of some type of fraud. Moreover, the percentage of articles retracted because of fraud is roughly ten times higher than it was in 1975. While some of this may be because of greater scrutiny, an increase of that magnitude should not be ignored, because the consequences of fraud in the medical literature can be devastating.

Consider two examples: The current movement against vaccination for children stemmed—in large part—from a well-publicized but fraudulent 1998 paper in the *Lancet*, one of Great Britain's top medical journals. In another case, as many as forty thousand women were treated for breast cancer with bone marrow transplants in the 1990s at a cost of billions of dollars. This treatment was based on studies revealed to be fraudulent. Bone marrow transplant, effective for certain blood disorders, turned out to be not only relatively ineffective for breast cancer but also often dangerous.

The medical establishment has been lax about policing the rise in conflicts of interest. Scrutiny by the medical profession is supposed to guarantee against outside conflicts, but hypocrisy is rife as many doctors receive generous payments from pharmaceutical concerns and device manufacturers while publishing scientific studies that can hardly be described as disinterested. Likewise, doctors accept payment from the government to develop important nationwide medical guidelines that often involve millions of dollars. And government, like the private sector, has its own agendas.

While this goes on, medical journal editors openly acknowledge that they cannot find article reviewers without any financial ties to private companies. Quite often the physician-authors being reviewed have significant conflicts of interests. Despite this, the medical community assures itself, and the public, that the value of this expertise outweighs any bias the conflicts bring to medical science. Even politicians are held to a higher standard, if only slightly.

More than ever, medical researchers aim for articles that will attract the mainstream press. The rush to get research to the public sometimes means short-circuiting rigorous scientific peer review. That can leave the review process in the hands of journalists unqualified or unwilling to interpret data and conclusions.

To illustrate the problem, John Bohannon, a Harvard biologist, created a fake study in 2014. Using a pseudonym, he and his colleagues deliberately ran a poorly designed "clinical trial" with subjects they recruited and randomly assigned to different diet regimens. They mined the results for anything that looked interesting and found that people lost weight 10 percent faster if they ate a chocolate bar every day. It was nothing more than a random finding. Yet the study was accepted by several online scientific journals within twenty-four hours, and the study was reported on the front page of Europe's largest daily newspaper. From there it went around the world via the Internet. Bohannon even concocted a cleverly designed news release to trumpet the findings. The results then appeared in magazines and on television in more than twenty countries. Ironically, only sharp-eyed online readers read the study critically. From the experience, Bohannon cautioned, "You have to know how to read a scientific paper—and actually bother to do it. . . . Hopefully our little experiment will make reporters and readers alike more skeptical."

There is no quick fix for the erosion of trust in medical studies. There have been calls for a new spate of bureaucratic rules or greater federal funding for investigative bodies. This is a quixotic quest; trust in science does not come from rules or money. Doctors and researchers must be taught early in their careers that intellectual honesty is more valuable than anything else, even personal advancement—*especially* personal advancement. Along with that, the general public must be better educated and display greater interest in science. Journalists should be trained to read and interpret medical studies and be willing to question research.

The fault is not in our stars but in ourselves. Admittedly, the long-term prospects for these remedies are not promising. Unfortunately, if the current trend continues, medical studies will become the "reality television" of science—difficult for outside observers to tell what has been manipulated and what hasn't.

31

COMPARATIVE EFFECTIVENESS RESEARCH: BUT WHAT IF THE RESEARCH DOESN'T SHOW WHAT YOU WANT?

One man's risky and over-priced treatment
is another man's income stream.

—HEALTH WRITER MAGGIE MAHAR

SEVERAL YEARS AGO, a congressional $787 billion economic stimulus package earmarked $1.1 billion to compare different medical treatments for specific illnesses. This "comparative effectiveness research" attempted to answer questions such as whether drugs or surgery work better in various medical conditions such as low back pain.

The impetus for this program, endorsed by President Obama during his 2008 campaign, was a growing skepticism voiced by health economists and policy experts who feel much of what doctors currently do is expensive and doesn't actually work. There is unquestionably much to be gained from such research. In many cases, surgical treatments haven't been randomized against nonsurgical therapy, and many drugs used in psychiatry haven't been evaluated comparatively against nonpharmacologic treatments. In addition there is insufficient follow-up on the long-term side effects of many approved drugs now on the market, and many medical devices used today haven't been sufficiently evaluated.

Comparative effectiveness research has generated great optimism in Washington. Representative Pete Stark (D-CA), former chairman of the Health Ways and Means subcommittee, summarized the optimism thusly: "The new research will eventually save money and lives." He explained that the United States spends over $1 trillion a year on health care and patients are put at risk, with billions of dollars spent each year on ineffective or unnecessary treatments, but "we have little information about which treatments work best for which patients." In a report accompanying the economic recovery package, the House Appropriations Committee echoed Stark's hopes by saying this research could "yield significant payoffs" because less effective, more expensive treatments "will no longer be prescribed."

Unfortunately, from a medical standpoint, these expectations often prove overconfident. It is foolish to predict the outcome of medical research in advance—the results may not be what we expect. We want cheaper therapies to be better, and in fact they often are. But in medicine, it simply doesn't follow that cheaper is automatically better. What then? What does the government do if research finds expensive back surgery turns out to be more effective than medication and physical therapy? What happens if long-term psychotherapy happens to be more effective at treating depression than short-term antidepressant therapy? What if cardiac surgery demonstrates it prolongs life for patients in their eighties and nineties? Will researchers feel subtle, unstated pressure, or even overt pressure, to gear studies that will result in findings that allow the government or insurers to limit coverage for expensive treatments?

This is a fundamental dilemma with large-scale, government-sponsored medical research. Quite often the results depend on who does the studies. The makeup of any proposed council of government advisers will likely have a major influence not only on the type of studies but on the actual findings of those studies. This is not a theoretical concern. European countries have faced this exact problem translating government-sponsored comparative effectiveness research into public policy.

Completely disinterested researchers are not always those selected to perform studies. Some scientists may feel political pressure to turn out the results sought by their patrons. Moreover, it's the rare specialist or surgeon who performs a study and acknowledges his or her specialty's approach is inferior to the alternative, especially if these findings have major financial implications for that specialty. Even then, professional specialty organizations are often loath to accept such findings. Anyone who doubts this need only consult the nearest medical library.

All of this is likely to result in warfare between strange bedfellows. Consumer groups, unions, employers, and insurers are likely to support government research efforts as a means of reducing waste (and cutting costs). The for-profit health care industry will find itself on the other side of the trenches since programs to make health care more efficient may be viewed as a threat to their economic well-being.

Despite the best efforts of our best scientists who do comparative effectiveness research, there will always be uncertainty in medical treatment. I hope that the economists, policy makers, and doctors remember that fact, since billions of dollars and the nation's health is at stake. They should heed Swedish physicians with extensive experience in comparative effectiveness research in Europe, who caution, "A decision to prioritize a less therapeutically effective medicine because of cost-based considerations over an effective, but more expensive, medicine could lead to some serious political, social and moral dilemmas."

32

THE EASIEST PERSON
TO FOOL IS YOURSELF

---

*This long history of learning how not to fool ourselves—
of having utter scientific integrity—is, I'm sorry to say,
something that we haven't specifically included in any particular
course that I know of. We just hope you've caught on by osmosis.*

—Richard Feynman to California Institute
of Technology graduates

SCIENTIFIC INTEGRITY IS THE THEME of the Greek tragedies that in the last decade or so involved two of America's most prestigious physicians. Both men worked for decades to reach the pinnacle of the medical profession; then both were brought low.

The first of the dramatis personae was octogenarian Dr. Sidney Gilman, chairman of neurology at the University of Michigan for over a quarter of a century from 1977 to 2004. A former professor at Harvard and Columbia and past president of the American Neurological Society, he authored hundreds of scientific papers, served on the editorial boards of key medical journals, and was a consultant to the Food and Drug Administration and several major pharmaceutical firms. Nearing the end of his chairmanship at Michigan, he was honored with the establishment of a neurology service at the university hospital and an annual lecture series, both named for him.

Then in 2014 Dr. Gilman found himself in a quite different role: key government witness in federal court. In a huge Wall Street insider trading trial, he admitted to providing confidential inside information about a new drug under development for Alzheimer's disease to the hedge fund portfolio manager who was the defendant in the trial. The hedge fund company realized over a quarter billion dollars from the information.

As chairman of the safety monitoring committee testing the Alzheimer's drug, Dr. Gilman was scheduled to present the study results at a scientific conference in Chicago. Twelve days before the conference, he deliberately leaked the results to the portfolio manager. The resulting stock transaction, and the relationship between Dr. Gilman and the defendant, attracted the attention of the Securities and Exchange Commission. The SEC subsequently indicted the manager and filed a complaint against Dr. Gilman. In exchange for avoiding prosecution, Dr. Gilman agreed to cooperate with the SEC investigation, testify in the trial, and pay nearly $250,000 to federal authorities. The affair forced him to resign his position at Michigan, and the institution severed its relationship with him. (The trader was ultimately convicted.)

Wayne State University law professor Peter Henning said the doctor may have been naive when savvy, big money Wall Street investors befriended him. Henning told the *Ann Arbor Observer*, "I don't believe he thought through the consequences of his actions, what a black mark they would leave on his career. I mean, this is going to be what's in the first paragraph of his obituary. . . . At one point he looked at the man in the mirror and convinced himself he wasn't doing anything all that wrong."

The second protagonist, in a separate case, was Dr. Charles Denham, a leader in the patient safety movement that has become the centerpiece of

American medicine. Dr. Denham's credentials were impeccable: He was a member of the President's Circle of the National Academies of Science and editor in chief of the *Journal of Patient Safety*, and he was associated with the Harvard School of Public Health and Mayo Clinic College of Medicine and Science. He has chaired the Safe Practices Program of the Leapfrog Group, a consortium of Fortune 500 companies with billions of dollars in health care purchasing power. The required reading periodical for all health care executives, *Modern Healthcare*, named him one of America's 50 Most Powerful Physician Executives several times.

His name also came up in the legal world in 2014 when the US Department of Justice accused a health care company, CareFusion Corp., of paying Dr. Denham $11.6 million in kickbacks while he served as cochair of a committee of the nonprofit National Quality Forum, which makes national practice recommendations on patient safety.

The Justice Department alleged the payments were meant to promote sales of a preoperative skin preparation and to market it for unapproved uses, in violation of the federal False Claims Act. In a public statement, a Justice Department spokesman said, "Corrupting the standard-setting process through kickbacks can affect the healthcare treatment choices that doctors and hospitals may make for patients." Dr. Denham, facing no charges, admitted to being paid the money but disagreed with the characterization of "kickback." CareFusion agreed to pay $40.1 million to resolve the allegations.

The medical community has been less than vigorous about policing these types of conflicts of interest. It strongly abjures trivial situations like pharmaceutical companies providing lunch for low-paid medical residents and students. Yet there is a remarkably laissez-faire attitude toward the potential bias of prominent physicians doing research for pharmaceutical firms or developing important nationwide medical guidelines, which may involve millions or even billions of dollars. A top university research physician recently confided to me that it is fairly common for physicians involved in drug trials and clinical guideline development to have significant conflicts of interest.

Every Greek tragedy has its chorus. In these particular cases, it is the late physicist Richard Feynman, one of the great scientists of the twentieth century and an avatar of scientific integrity. Feynman, a Nobel Prize winner, was the man who demonstrated the cause of the space shuttle *Challenger* explosion in a simple experiment on national television and was highly critical of the intellectual honesty of many involved in the project. He continually emphasized that scientific integrity is a principle of scientific thought that demands utmost honesty—in essence, leaning over backward intellectually to be honest. The Gilman and Denham cases suggest that in today's medical environment, this approach is in jeopardy.

Forty-four years ago, giving the California Institute of Technology commencement address, Feynman made a timeless observation about scientific integrity: "The first principle is that you must not fool yourself—and you are the easiest person to fool. So you have to be very careful about that."

33

PHYSICIAN, HEAL THYSELF

---

*The biggest danger here is that it leaves a cloud over the patients
and their families over whether they were put at some unnecessary
risk. All of those questions are in their heads. . . .
When money is inserted into the equation, there is no trust.*

—US DISTRICT JUDGE SHARON JOHNSON COLEMAN,
PRESIDING OVER A 2016 KICKBACK TRIAL

IS THE PSYCHIATRIC PROFESSION, and medicine in general, sinking
in an ethical swamp? With greater scrutiny devoted to pharmaceutical
companies' payments to doctors, psychiatrists appear high on the list of
beneficiaries among all medical specialties. Financial arrangements between
psychiatrists and drug companies may be a factor in the recent rise in antipsychotic drug expenses for Medicaid programs, as well as the increasing
use of expensive antipsychotic drugs, especially for children. The enormity
of the conflict of interest problem is highlighted by three high-profile cases
involving influential psychiatrists and large payments from the pharmaceutical industry.

The first case involved a weekly public radio program dealing with psychiatric issues and mental disorders, *The Infinite Mind*, heard in over three hundred markets with more than one million listeners. A congressional investigation revealed the psychiatrist who hosted the program, Dr. Frederick K. Goodwin, earned at least $1.3 million between 2000 and 2007 by giving marketing lectures for pharmaceutical firms, income that was never disclosed on the program. The companies who paid him often had a significant financial interest in subjects discussed on the show.

Dr. Goodwin received more than $300,000 in one year for promotional lectures dealing with medications that were frequent topics of discussion on *The Infinite Mind*. He rationalized the conflict of interest by blaming a change in the ethical environment for misunderstandings about his consulting arrangements. "It didn't occur to me that my doing what every other expert in the field does might be considered a conflict of interest." (An NPR spokesman said that had they been aware of Dr. Goodwin's financial interests, they would not have aired the program, and they removed the program from their satellite radio service.)

A second case was that of Dr. Charles Nemeroff, a prominent Emory University psychiatrist and the principal investigator for drug treatment studies of depression for the National Institutes of Health. He received over $2 million in consulting fees from the pharmaceutical companies involved in those studies. Although Nemeroff, as chairman of psychiatry at Emory, signed university documents pledging to accept no more than $10,000 a year from a single company, according to congressional investigators, he allegedly received payment far in excess of that. He voluntarily stepped down as chairman of the psychiatry department at Emory.

The third case involved Dr. Joseph Biederman, a leading child psychiatrist at Harvard Medical School and Massachusetts General Hospital. Biederman, a particularly influential figure in the field of bipolar disorders in children, worked in concert with a drug company that provided nearly $1 million to establish a research center at Massachusetts General. The center, besides aiding children with psychiatric disorders, had as one of its publicly stated goals to advance the commercial goals of the drug company. In addition Biederman neglected to disclose to Harvard over $1 million that he received from the pharmaceutical industry, a violation of Harvard's disclosure policies.

Relationships between physicians and the pharmaceutical industry are an essential arrangement in the development and testing of new medications. Drug development would be impossible without physician input. But large payments to high-profile, influential physicians, especially when the payments are not disclosed to the public, raise serious questions. Are the recommendations these physicians provide to the medical community of newer, more costly medications made at the expense of nondrug therapy, generic drugs, and older, less expensive medications that may be equally effective?

In fairness to psychiatrists, they are not alone in this ethical morass. Cardiologists and many surgical subspecialties have become entangled in similar conflict of interest problems. The role of the "expert" physician as respected authority has made them an attractive target of the pharmaceutical industry. Insurance company restrictions, the consumer-based medicine movement, the Internet, relaxed restrictions on direct patient marketing, and the emphasis on practice guidelines by expert committees have all reduced the influence of individual physicians and their prescribing patterns. Big pharma realizes the bang for their promotional buck lies with prominent physicians who are professional leaders.

Will the medical profession pass the point of no return? Federal oversight and more disclosure rules are necessary but not sufficient. The government's role, especially in private industry, is limited, and many times professional disclosure rules have simply permitted physicians to accept large payments as long as they are disclosed, in effect sanctioning ethically dubious arrangements.

If physicians are to retain the public confidence and maintain their own integrity, it will require a commitment by both professional leaders and the rank and file to create more ombudsmen in the medical community, a role currently assumed by a small vocal minority. Physician, heal thyself—at stake is the soul of the medical profession.

34

SIGNPOST UP AHEAD:
GOOD INTENTIONS

Hell is paved with good intentions, not bad ones.
All men mean well.

—GEORGE BERNARD SHAW

BENEFICENCE, the desire to do kind deeds, is the fundamental principle at the heart of medicine. Yet one of the painful lessons medicine teaches is that good intentions don't always lead to good outcomes. Occasionally, the result of good intentions is terrible tragedy. Two separate medical incidents, one involving the Food and Drug Administration (FDA) and antidepressants and the other involving the United Nations Children's Fund (UNICEF) and contaminated drinking water, are painful reminders of the lesson of unintended consequences.

In the past two decades, several large population studies have demonstrated an association, but not necessarily a cause and effect, between certain antidepressants and suicidal ideation/behavior in youths. Because patients who receive antidepressants have a higher risk of suicide than the general population, the studies were unable to establish conclusive causation attributed to the medications. The question remains: Were observed suicides the result of the prescribed medicines or the underlying condition? The FDA, acting in good faith, elected to issue a requirement that a black box warning, advising of a potential suicide risk, be placed on antidepressants prescribed for youths and young adults.

Several studies have suggested the black box warnings may have had the unintended consequence of placing more youths at risk of suicide. Researchers found the black box warnings resulted in a reduction in antidepressant prescriptions for adolescents and adults. They demonstrated an increase in youth suicides associated with the temporal decline in the use of antidepressants, a finding that may have also occurred in the Netherlands after a similar warning about antidepressant drugs was issued there.

One study author, Hendricks Brown, said, "The overall effect of these newer antidepressants is very likely that they reduce suicide risk considerably. Overall, the new antidepressants provide a large protective benefit. If there is any group of people who are adversely affected by taking these antidepressants, it has to be a very small group." Brown said health policy decisions are sometimes based on limited information, and the FDA might have inadvertently placed more youth at risk by mandating the warnings. The issue of youth suicide and its causes is incredibly complex, especially in the era of social media. While the FDA was understandably cautious with its black box warning and beneficence was the goal, it may have been an example of good intentions gone wrong.

An even more tragic instance of unintended consequences was highlighted in 2010 in the *Lancet*. It involved what is believed to be the largest known case of mass poisoning in world history. In the early 1970s, the newly formed country of Bangladesh, formerly East Pakistan, was ravaged by a cyclone, famines, and political unrest. Much of the world first found out about the plight of the suffering populace when Beatle George Harrison organized the Concert for Bangladesh, the first charity rock concert.

At the time, the only drinking water available to most Bangladeshis came from ponds and shallow pits contaminated by human and agricultural waste. Diarrhea, cholera, and typhoid were rampant and killed thousands, especially children, every year. Western relief organizations headed by UNICEF embarked on a large-scale program to help Bangladesh by drilling millions of shallow tube wells that provided drinking water by hand pump.

The tube well drilling program drastically reduced the spread of gastrointestinal diseases and cut child mortality in half. For this it was hailed worldwide, but what no one realized at the time was that the groundwater feeding many of those tube wells contained extremely high concentrations of arsenic. The naturally occurring arsenic, leached from rocks as the result of runoff from Himalayan snows, could not be detected when the wells were dug. Millions of the Bangladeshis have been poisoned with the highly toxic, carcinogenic chemical for three decades as a result of the wells drilled in the 1970s.

Programs are currently underway to test for arsenic and dig deeper wells that tap safe groundwater, but Dr. Joseph Graziano, health professor at Columbia University, explained, "Bangladesh's drinking water is one of the world's most hazardous because of the presence of arsenic. An estimated 40 million people, roughly 30 percent of the population, are currently exposed to poisonous levels of arsenic." Government efforts to reduce the arsenic exposure have been only partially successful, and millions still consume tainted water.

As these cases indicate, medical decision-making is a balancing act of risk and benefit. Decisions come with hidden variables and unknown facts. Unfortunately, this means some risks are poorly perceived. The familiar adage "the road to hell is paved with good intentions" may be an overstatement, but occasionally the signpost marked GOOD INTENTIONS leads down a tragic path. The safe road turns out to be filled with danger.

35

CONCUSSION AND CONFLICT
OF INTEREST

It's just business. Nothing personal.

—Various sources

IN A REVEALING SCENE from the 2015 movie *Concussion*, former Pittsburgh Steeler team physician Dr. Julian Bailes, played by Alec Baldwin, and county coroner Dr. Cyril Wecht, played by Albert Brooks, examine pathology slides of the brain of a retired player who died presumably as a result of repeated head trauma. Bailes explains to Wecht that National Football League (NFL) team physicians must administer all sorts of drugs to players, from painkillers to antidepressants, in order to keep them playing.

An outraged Wecht says disapprovingly, "It's not medicine."

Bailes explains, "It's business."

Concussion is based on the true story of Dr. Bennet Omalu, played by Will Smith, the forensic pathologist who discovered a unique type of brain damage, chronic traumatic encephalopathy (CTE), in several NFL players who died after retirement. The movie depicts a situation in which the NFL attempts to suppress Dr. Omalu's findings, the implication being that the league had a conflict of interest because admitting the dangers of head trauma while playing football would be bad for business.

The movie is well done, but, typical of today's Hollywood movies, there is little nuance in motives: Characters are either good (Omalu and his colleagues) or evil (the NFL and their representatives). Unlike real life, there is little middle ground.

One way the movie identifies the villains is that they are the ones with conflicts of interest—it's about business. A former NFL commissioner (bad guy) is identified as having worked for a law firm that defends big tobacco. A player on the NFL compensation committee (bad guy) is called a "sell-out" by a player who was denied a settlement for his injuries. (That player on the compensation committee happened to be former Chicago Bear Dave Duerson, who later committed suicide, and his family has objected to how he is portrayed in the film.) In the movie, Dr. Bailes (good guy) is redeemed when he leaves his position as an NFL team physician and joins Dr. Omalu's side.

But movies "based on true stories" don't necessarily tell the whole truth. While Dr. Omalu did identify CTE in football players, he did not give the condition its name, as the movie claims. It was identified and named in boxers decades ago by earlier physicians. That is trivial.

More important, scientists, including in this case Dr. Omalu, often have significant conflicts of interest as well.

The brain findings Dr. Omalu described were all postmortem, and there is currently no way to identify CTE before death. Consequently, there are tremendous medical and financial incentives to discover a test that will demonstrate findings of CTE in living patients. And Dr. Omalu is a partner in a company that proposes to do exactly that. The company, Taumark, owns exclusive rights to a radioactive compound that, when injected into the bloodstream, is supposed to show up in brain scans and identify CTE.

If successful, the test would be extremely expensive, and the demand would be tremendous.

In 2013 after an initial study of five NFL players, Taumark was deluged by demands from professional athletes and the parents of amateur football players. Unfortunately, right now the technique remains an experimental research tool. Independent experts caution that it has no proven clinical value at present. "The whole field is in a very early state since we don't even know what CTE is," said Dr. Douglas Smith, a traumatic brain injury researcher at the University of Pennsylvania. "Instead of having everybody in a mad dash to get a scan, we need to vet these tests so they are validated."

This did not deter two of Dr. Omalu's partners from issuing unfounded claims on the company website stating, "Despite the devastating conse- quence of traumatic brain injury and the large number of athletes, military personnel and other head trauma victims at risk, until now, no method has been developed for early detection or tracking of the brain pathology associated with these injuries." Shortly after that, the FDA, which has not approved Taumark's compound for clinical use, forced them to remove that claim. The compound has yet to prove specific for CTE.

Preventing and detecting brain injury in athletes is a huge emerging industry, and Dr. Omalu's company could reap immense profits (although other companies have begun testing their own compounds). While his com- pany goes about raising millions of start-up dollars, he is notably reticent about the details of going forward. He told a Pittsburgh interviewer, "It's a business. I cannot reveal the corporate plans. . . . When people say 'for-profit business,' I don't want people to say that as a derogatory [term]. . . . No, it is something good."

It certainly might be. There is nothing illegal about medical research- ers partnering in commercial ventures. As for being unethical, these types of relationships are encouraged by virtually every American university, so much so that issues of conflicts of interest are often glossed over. When I taught medical ethics to students and residents, they saw no problem with doctors partnering, although they were nearly unanimous that it was unethical if politicians did something similar.

As a Taumark partner, Dr. Omalu has an undeniable interest in the successful outcome of his company's brain trauma research. In no way does this mean Taumark's work will automatically be biased or invalid. But it does mean there will inevitably be questions about Dr. Omalu's credibility and even his integrity, which was depicted as unimpeachable in *Concussion*.

As Dr. Bailes observed, "It's business."

36

I AIN'T AFRAID OF NO MEDICAL GHOSTWRITERS

It was my fault. I should have read it before it came out.
—CHARLES BARKLEY ABOUT HIS AUTOBIOGRAPHY

HOW COULD YOU be misquoted in your own autobiography? Well, it happened to basketball-player-turned-broadcaster Charles Barkley, who gave the matter a simple explanation. In all likelihood, the problem was that Sir Charles employed a ghostwriter, nothing to be ashamed of since it puts him in decent company with the likes of Ronald Reagan (Robert Lindsey) and David Beckham (Tom Watt).

Athletes, politicians, and celebrities are often short on time, not to mention writing ability, and while they may be reluctant to admit it, ghostwriters are indispensable to telling their stories. But what's commonplace in the publishing industry has permeated the medical profession. In what has become a widespread practice, ghostwriters are substituting for doctors by writing articles for medical journals about important research. In some cases, it has reached the level of outright deception. The Senate Finance Committee investigated "medical ghostwriting" as part of its examination of pharmaceutical company influence on the health care industry. During the probe Senator Charles Grassley (R-IA) was given internal company documents showing that pharmaceutical giant Wyeth hired ghostwriters to write favorable medical journal articles about one of its widely marketed drugs.

According to the documents, a decade ago Wyeth developed in-house concepts for medical articles and hired a company that employs medical authors, who are not doctors, to write the manuscripts. Wyeth then recruited prestigious physicians to put their names on the articles as authors. Once the articles were ready, they were submitted to medical journals as if the doctors had written them. None of this was disclosed to the journals' editors or readers.

Medical ghostwriting has been an embarrassing issue before. *JAMA: The Journal of the American Medical Association* revealed that Merck had research studies prepared and written by nonphysician ghostwriters before arranging to have academic physicians put their names on the articles as authors. Recruited authors were frequently listed as primary authors and paid for their participation. Some manuscripts about the pain medication Vioxx were prepared by unacknowledged ghostwriters and attributed to prestigious physicians, who failed to disclose their payments from the company. (In an unrelated matter, Vioxx became the subject of lawsuits and was pulled from the market.) Merck has acknowledged that on occasion it hires outside medical writers to assist the doctors whose names eventually appear on the articles. It maintains the doctors do contribute research and analysis and sign off on the final draft of all articles.

None of this means that published medical research is necessarily inaccurate or biased. Most articles are approved by independent peer review before publication. But it does raise questions for both the scientific and lay communities about the process of medical authorship and the integrity of everyone involved, including physicians who market their names and reputations posing as authors for articles they simply have not written.

The problem is the result of the increasing complexity of medical research. Today medical studies, whether they come from universities or private industry, involve teams of researchers including investigators, statisticians, and writers. In the case of pharmaceutical companies, where there are large sums of money at stake in new drug development and approval, the actual credits for a final paper, if published, might resemble those of a major motion picture.

Unfortunately, many physicians today have neither the time nor the training to write the type of prose necessary to publish these studies. The process of training doctors is in part to blame. Most medical students no longer take writing courses as undergraduates or in medical school. Whereas medical journals were once filled with doctors' entertaining, well-written accounts, journals today are filled with dense, turgid articles incomprehensible to outsiders (and not infrequently to those in the field).

Enter the medical ghostwriter. Most are professionally trained writers with a scientific background. Of course, as in any field, there are shills among them, but the majority are proud of their contribution to advancing the quality of medical research. Without them, many studies simply would not get published. But full disclosure is the key to ending the current deception. The ghosts must be expunged, and to do so, pharmaceutical companies and physicians must identify those people who actually write the words for them. In addition, as an editorial in *JAMA* noted, "[Medical] journal editors also bear some of the responsibility for enabling companies to manipulate publications."

Conflicts of interest are a serious problem in the medical profession today, but ghostwriting is not necessarily a bad thing—when acknowledged and openly identified. The professional approach to medical ghostwriting should be that of the *Ghostbusters* theme—"I ain't afraid of no ghosts." Even if it is a double negative no self-respecting ghostwriter would ever tolerate.

37

THE BLACKEST
OF ALL BLACK MARKETS

If you think people are inherently good,
get rid of the police for 24 hours and see what happens.

—SYLVESTER STALLONE

SNOPES IS A WEBSITE specializing in investigating urban myths. It turns out Walt Disney wasn't cryogenically frozen after death, and a tooth left in a glass of Coca-Cola won't dissolve overnight. But the site also investigates more sinister urban myths like the one about people who reportedly have been drugged and had a kidney removed against their will as part of a black market in transplantable organs.

The website diligently tracks the myth's origins, its perpetuation (including on a 1991 episode of *Law & Order*), and in a detailed, responsible fashion, debunks the story. There is only one problem—at least in South Asia, the story is not an urban myth. In 2008 an organ transplant ring working out of several Indian states victimized indigent day laborers in poor sections of India. Authorities believe hundreds of people had their kidneys removed and then sold to clients who traveled to India from around the world. A police raid on a covert clinic near New Delhi uncovered a kidney transplant waiting list with forty-eight names, including those of several foreigners (known as "medical tourists"). The police suspect the ring involved doctors, nurses, hospitals, paramedics, and a car outfitted as a tissue matching laboratory. Bioethicists have long suspected organs have also been harvested from prisoners condemned to death in Communist China.

While nothing remotely like this has happened in the United States (although at least two American citizens may have been on the police's recovered client list in India), this organ black market is an ominous development. The sale of an organ is currently illegal in the United States, with bioethics groups, transplant organizations, and the Vatican all inveighing against putting a concrete price on a kidney. Citing a host of abuses, they envision the exploitation of the poor who might opt for quick cash, as well as recipients reneging on payment agreements, shoddy postoperative care for poor donors, and ultimately the urban myth that has become real in India: a black market in organs.

But there are nearly seventy-five thousand domestic patients with renal failure waiting for kidneys, and each year several thousand of them die before receiving a kidney. Consequently, there is a growing movement in the United States to commodify organs—expand the pool of available organs by offering compensation to people to donate a kidney (a person can live with one healthy kidney). Supporters have proposed changes in the law, including a regulated free market in organs (an "incentive system"), which might save the lives of some of those who currently die awaiting donor organs. They claim a well-regulated federal incentive system would actually prevent a black market of exploited donors. A Nobel Prize–winning economist has even calculated a price he claims would eliminate the current waiting list.

Without putting a price on a kidney, the organ-donation system needs streamlining. Simply relying on altruism, however commendable, does not provide for the number of kidneys needed to eliminate long and sometimes fatal waiting times. The federal government should provide new incentives such as significant tax credits and the assumption of long-term health care costs for those willing to donate a kidney. A radical idea worth discussing—once they have given their gift, perhaps those who donate a kidney should never have to pay either income tax or for their health care. Such a plan would not necessarily mean lost revenue for the government since thousands currently disabled by renal failure would then be able to return to work.

But absolute faith in the free market corrupts absolutely. When kidneys or other organs become simply another commodity, there will be no shortage of those willing to exploit others. That's why in addition to providing added incentives for organ donation, the federal government should reinforce its vigilance against the unauthorized procurement and sale of organs in light of the Indian experience.

The problem of how to encourage organ donation illustrates an eternal medical dilemma—the conflicting role money plays in health care. The quest for profit drives the research and technology that provide immeasurable benefit to American patients. But the naked edge of the free market also invites exploitation, fraud, and crime, even in medicine. International trafficking in transplantable organs would be the worst conceivable black market. And that's no urban myth.

38

DOPED: PERFORMANCE-ENHANCING DRUGS KEEP WINNING THE RACE AGAINST TESTING

The drug problem has always been with us, and it always will be. Athletes have always used performance-enhancing substances. . . . It's human nature to try to obtain every possible advantage for success. If there were a drug available that would dramatically increase the ability of university faculty to get grants, you'd better believe they'd be injecting their butts with it in front of Old Main.

—CHARLES YESALIS, MPH, LEADING EXPERT ON
PERFORMANCE-ENHANCING DRUGS

THE HISTORY OF ATHLETES using performance-enhancing drugs (PEDs) goes back at least two thousand years, when ancient Greek athletes used mushrooms and opioids during athletic competitions, including the first Olympic Games. There are reports of European cyclists using a variety of stimulants during the late nineteenth century. In the twentieth century, German physicians discovered the first injectable anabolic steroids, and these drugs, along with amphetamines, may have been administered to Nazi troops during World War II. After the war, use of these drugs took off in both amateur and professional sporting events.

The drug situation became a reflection of the Cold War—drug use a symbol of the political competition between the East and West. Soviet weight lifters achieved great success in the 1950s using anabolic steroids. While the first Olympic drug testing was established in 1968, the world's attention was drawn to the incredible performances of East German female swimmers in the 1970s. Many of these young women were selected by the government from an early age, taken from their families, and received intensive training and sophisticated chemical regimens, leaving them with terrible physical and psychological complications years later. Some are infertile or have given birth to deformed children. Others have developed male sex characteristics, and at least one developed so many male sex characteristics, she underwent a sex-change operation.

When East Germany collapsed, these swimmers' unfortunate stories were revealed, and the world took note of the drug problem in sports. Meanwhile in the West, European cyclists used amphetamines routinely in the 1960s. In the United States, PEDs made their way into professional sports. In 1970 former New York Yankees pitcher Jim Bouton wrote *Ball Four*, a bestseller about his life in baseball, describing widespread use of amphetamines, known as "greenies."

Gradually, medical advances made PEDs more accessible to professional athletes, and drug testing could not keep pace with the drug explosion. In the last two decades, drug use has proliferated. Top Olympians, including Marion Jones and Ben Johnson, tested positive for banned compounds, calling their world-class performances into question. Johnson, once "the world's fastest man," had his world record one-hundred-meter dash time thrown out and was temporarily banned from his sport. Jones, among

America's top Olympians, was stripped of five Olympic medals and went to jail for events revolving around her use of illegal PEDs.

Following his career, former Oakland Athletics outfielder Jose Canseco publicly charged that steroid use was widespread in baseball. His accusations were first viewed skeptically, but as baseball performances reached new heights, some players confessed to using drugs, lending Canseco's claims credibility. In 2005 Congress held public hearings, and players including Mark McGwire and Sammy Sosa, hailed as heroes only several years before, were unconvincing in their denials of steroid use. It's been disclosed that stars including Alex Rodriguez, Barry Bonds, Andy Pettite, Manny Ramirez, and David Ortiz have all tested positive for PEDs at some point in their careers.

Meanwhile, the abuse of PEDs has crept into college and high school athletics. Surveys indicate more than one million American children between the ages of twelve and seventeen have taken PEDs (including creatine, which falls into a special category). It would be naive to believe the success of professional athletes who have used PEDs has not influenced younger athletes. Since testing is expensive and sometimes impractical at the lower levels, no one knows how serious the problem is. However, the accessibility of these drugs through the Internet and other channels makes PEDs a serious public health issue at all levels of sports.

What are we talking about when we say PEDs? The term is all encompassing and nonspecific. It includes some legal drugs and others that are illegal. Some of the drugs are injected, some taken orally, and others used in skin patches. It includes naturally occurring substances, synthetic compounds, drugs used for other legitimate purposes, nutritional supplements, and drugs used not for performance but to mask or counter the effects of other drugs. This is why it is hard to draw absolute medical conclusions about what drugs athletes ingest.

Many athletes distrust the scientific community on the issue of PEDs. Much of the early scientific literature stated unequivocally that certain commonly used compounds like anabolic steroids did not improve performance and routinely caused dramatic side effects. This ran directly counter to the underground athletic community experience and had the effect of discrediting the medical literature. Athletes and their trainers experimented with multiple drug combinations and dosing regimens that were based outside mainstream pharmacology. This information was eventually transmitted by word of mouth to others, who modified what they heard and created their own regimens. Physicians were generally unaware of how the compounds were being used and rarely performed tests reflecting real-life situations. Even today, reliable knowledge about the benefits and dangers of PEDs remains hard to come by in the medical literature. There is a small cadre of experts working diligently to answer these questions, but there's an ongoing development of new drugs and methods of administration.

The following discussion is an admittedly incomplete overview of the medical effects of PEDs and is based on the current status of medical knowledge about commonly used compounds.

Anabolic Steroids

These PEDs are derivatives of the male hormone testosterone. *Anabolic* refers to their ability to stimulate protein synthesis and increase muscle mass. Not all steroids are anabolic. Anabolic steroids should not be confused with corticosteroids such as prednisone, which are commonly used in sports. Corticosteroids are generally injected into injured tissue to suppress short-term inflammation. While their use is sometimes controversial in the management of injury, corticosteroids are generally not considered PEDs.

Anabolic steroids include injectable drugs such as testosterone and nandrolone and oral drugs such as stanozolol. These drugs can be used for short periods of time or in on-off cycles of six to twelve weeks, a process known as stacking. Occasionally athletes will increase the dose significantly during a stacking cycle—this is known as pyramiding. Anabolic steroids basically build muscle mass, increasing size and strength, although users must train and eat properly to realize the greatest effect. Their benefit is obvious for power sports, such as weight lifting, wrestling, and football, but they may also benefit those who require bursts of energy, such as sprinters. For baseball players they have the obvious benefits of increasing strength, bat speed, and probably throwing velocity. It's possible they increase hand-eye coordination. There are other less measurable, but just as practical, competitive effects, such as increasing confidence and aggression. These are potent drugs with significant side effects, and a number of studies suggest they may be addictive, though the potential for addiction is a matter of debate.

In children they are especially dangerous since they accelerate the maturation process and result in growth plate closure and shortened adult height. In both children and adults, muscle growth may outstrip tendon and ligament support and result in increased injuries. In adults potential complications include cardiovascular disease (hypertension, accelerated atherosclerosis, heart attacks, heart failure), liver problems (hepatitis, liver tumors), endocrine problems (high blood sugar, decreased sexual characteristics and sperm production in men, masculinization in women), acne, and psychological changes (depression, irritability).

The exact incidence of complications is unknown since it is difficult to test these drugs under actual conditions. In addition since long-term experience is limited, it's unknown what happens in later life to young athletes using these drugs. Another important complication is the consequence of needle injection. Those who inject steroids are susceptible to serious and well-documented complications, including bacterial and chemical skin abscesses, viral hepatitis, HIV infection, and other serious blood infections.

Anabolic steroids are currently classified as Schedule III—they can only be obtained with a prescription. Possession of anabolic steroids without a prescription carries legal penalties, and unlawful distribution is a more serious legal offense. The International Olympic Committee (IOC) and most professional sports leagues in North America and Europe ban their use.

Steroid Precursors or Prohormones

These are hormones produced in the body that are ultimately converted to testosterone. Two common precursors are dehydroepiandrosterone (DHEA) and androstenedione (the drug baseball player Mark McGwire admitted taking). These drugs have no specific medical indication and technically are not anabolic steroids. Because they are converted to anabolic steroids in the body, they have similar effects and side effects, though they are relatively less potent than actual anabolic steroids. Since they were classified differently than anabolic steroids for many years, they were popular ingredients in nutritional supplements. However, the federal government has reclassified these drugs in the same category as anabolic steroids, and there are penalties at the federal level for possession and distribution. Androstenedione was a popular supplement in Major League Baseball until it was banned in 2004. It's also banned by the IOC, National Football League (NFL), and National Collegiate Athletic Association (NCAA).

Human Growth Hormone

Human growth hormone (HGH) is a naturally occurring hormone of the pituitary gland. It is used to treat patients with certain growth disorders who are deficient in its production and is used in some specific chronic diseases. It is a popular PED today because it can't be detected by most routine testing procedures. Its effects on normal subjects are unclear although there are reports it increases strength and decreases body fat. Former Chicago White Sox pitcher Jim Parque admitted to injecting HGH after an injury while an active major leaguer. (It was not banned at the time.) His experience is instructive; he describes that it did not make him stronger but allowed him to train harder because it shortened recovery time between workouts. The capacity for drugs such as HGH to permit users longer, more rigorous training sessions and to shorten recovery time after workouts should not be underestimated. That is an important, albeit indirect, factor in performance enhancement.

The side effects of HGH can be serious and include diabetes, heart disease, arthritis, and skeletal abnormalities, including jaw prominence and skull enlargement. Until recently most HGH was collected from cadavers, and use of the drug carried the risk of viral disease transmission. Today HGH is made synthetically, eliminating this danger and making it more accessible to patients and athletes. HGH is legal with a prescription, but distribution without a prescription can lead to a fine and/or prison term. Many "HGH creams and sprays" are available through the Internet, but they are most likely worthless since the body can only use HGH when it is injected.

Blood Doping

Blood doping is a technique especially popular with competitive cyclists and long-distance runners. It involves increasing the number of oxygen-carrying red blood cells in the body in order to increase aerobic performance. Formerly, athletes would store their own blood and receive it as transfusions near the time of competition. Today the same effect can be obtained through the administration of erythropoietin (EPO), an agent that stimulates red blood cell production (used in patients with chronic renal failure who are anemic). Recently it has been demonstrated that in certain types of brain injury, EPO has protective effects that are independent of its red blood cell stimulation. The mechanism of this "neuroprotective" effect is uncertain, and it may also play a role in the benefits that athletes realize by using EPO.

EPO is difficult to detect with current testing. Blood doping, while it increases aerobic capability, is extremely dangerous. Increasing the number of red blood cells in the body essentially makes blood thicker and can result in heart attacks, strokes, and sudden death. These complications are more common in athletes who become dehydrated. Since 1987 the deaths of at least eighteen Belgian and Dutch cyclists have been attributed to EPO. Interestingly training at high altitudes for long periods of time, while controversial, can result in the same effect as blood doping—that is, increasing red blood cell numbers and aerobic potential by stimulating the natural production of EPO.

Stimulants

The use of stimulants as PEDs ranges from caffeine to ephedrine and its derivatives to amphetamines. Unlike hormones, these drugs don't increase strength or aerobic capabilities. They can be effective because they reduce the sense of fatigue, increase alertness, heighten euphoria, and lessen the sensation of pain.

Caffeine is the most commonly used drug by athletes. In moderation it may increase endurance and improve performance. When used excessively, it may interfere with athletic performance and cause dehydration. Olympic and NCAA competition permit caffeine up to certain levels (roughly the amount in six cups of coffee over twenty-four hours). Higher levels are banned. Ephedrine and its derivatives are commonly used asthma drugs that have been used as PEDs. They stimulate the nervous system, although their effect on athletic performance is unclear. (Bodybuilders claim they increase energy, metabolism, and training drive and help mobilize body fat.) In 2003 an ephedrine derivative was linked to the death of Steve Bechler, a prospective pitcher for the Baltimore Orioles.

Most studies have demonstrated little athletic benefit to these drugs. A number of deaths and cardiovascular complications have been reported with the use of ephedrine and related compounds, especially in hot weather. Ephedrine-like compounds represent a lucrative export industry from China. Compounds such as ma huang and similar dietary supplements have been touted to improve muscle tone and energy levels, although there is little documentation. Ephedrine and its derivatives remain legal in the United States under certain conditions; however, the

Food and Drug Administration (FDA) has banned many supplements containing ephedrine.

The IOC, NCAA, and NFL have all banned ephedrine-containing compounds. Amphetamines were once a popular drug of abuse in sports, especially in baseball because of the grueling daily schedule. Amphetamine derivatives have some therapeutic uses in conditions such as attention deficit disorder. They are also used as recreational drugs, as well as reportedly by students as a study aid and in the military by pilots on long missions. The dangers of amphetamines are well known, and their use was banned in Major League Baseball in 2006.

Other Drugs

Certain drugs with legitimate therapeutic uses are also used either as PEDs or to mask the signs and symptoms of the drugs mentioned above. Inderal, a beta blocker, is a commonly used cardiovascular agent that also decreases hand tremor and reduces anxiety by blocking the effects of adrenalin. It is used in such sports as archery and riflery. (Musicians, singers, and public speakers also employ it because it minimizes stage fright.) It has been banned by the IOC because of the advantage it confers by reducing tremors.

Diuretics are used for rapid weight loss and occasionally as masking agents in an attempt to beat drug tests by diluting the urine. Therapeutic hormones such as clomiphene and human chorionic gonadotropin (HCG) have been used to stimulate recovery after anabolic steroid cycling.

Creatine and Other Supplements

Dietary supplements, products containing substances such as vitamins, minerals, botanicals, and amino acids, are meant to supplement normal oral intake. Creatine may be the most widely used supplement in the United States. In 2000 creatine accounted for more than $400 million in sales. Creatine is a naturally occurring compound stored in skeletal muscle. It is essentially muscle protein and is available by eating meat or fish. It's then synthesized and stored in the body. Creatine supplements are basically larger, more concentrated amounts of this muscle protein.

Creatine is taken to increase muscle mass and enhance performance. The compound has been studied in different types of athletic activity, and there are indications it improves performance in certain types of high-intensity exercise, especially running and jumping. This effect has not been seen in all types of aerobic activity and may depend on factors including the athlete's body mass and training regimen. Creatine appears to increase weight and decrease body fat in the short term, although much of the weight increase may be due to water retention. Also it is unclear whether short-term increases in muscle mass are an anabolic effect or the result of increased training.

Is creatine dangerous? The answer is unclear. While there are anec-dotal reports of significant problems, current literature seems to indicate that when creatine is taken in recommended doses, there is no definitive evidence of serious harm. This doesn't mean there is no risk or that the product can be deemed completely safe. In addition little is known about possible long-term effects of chronic creatine use. At present, creatine, if taken, is best used under the auspices of a qualified trainer or physician familiar with the compound.

Other supplements abound, especially those containing supernormal amounts of basic dietary amino acids. While there are often glowing claims that these supplements improve performance and release endogenous hor-mones, the vast majority of these claims are unsubstantiated and probably have no validity. Many supplements offer nothing more than a high-priced, well-balanced diet. They may be safe but are probably ineffective and are very expensive. It should be remembered that the FDA can't rigorously examine every product on the market, and there may be counterfeit prod-ucts (especially through the Internet or imported from abroad) prepared in an unsterile manner or tainted with substances such as anabolic steroids. This may be a source of positive drug tests for athletes uncertain of what is in the products they use. Ultimately, athletes are responsible for what they put in their bodies.

This is only a partial list of the PEDs and supplements currently available. But new designer drugs are being developed constantly. Little is known of these new drugs—even those designing these drugs are often working by trial and error.

Charles Yesalis, an expert on drug use in athletes, has observed that it is human nature for individuals to seek every advantage in competition, and athletes are among the most competitive individuals. The race is always on to look for better drugs and ways to beat testing. The tests will improve, but testers will always remain one step behind users—the entire exercise resembles a high-tech game of cops and robbers. All too often we extol the virtues of, rather than condemn, athletes who use these drugs.

We put undue emphasis on winning at all costs and transmit this to our athletes, who believe they must use these drugs to succeed. This is especially dangerous in the case of children, who feel the pressure even more acutely than adults and are at the greatest risk from these drugs. As one world-class cyclist so aptly put it, "What goes around comes around eventually. It can be 10 years, 15 years; it all comes out in the wash and where are you? A gold medal isn't as gold anymore."

39

A PILL NOT IN THE BEST INTERESTS OF HEALTHY STUDENTS

Canst thou not minister to a mind diseased,
Pluck from the memory a rooted sorrow,
Raze out the written troubles of the brain,
And with some sweet oblivious antidote
Cleanse the stuffed bosom of that perilous stuff
Which weighs upon the heart?

—WILLIAM SHAKESPEARE, *MACBETH*

SHOULD DOCTORS PRESCRIBE powerful stimulant drugs to improve the grades of underperforming but otherwise healthy schoolchildren? According to the *New York Times*, a pediatrician in Georgia, Dr. Michael Anderson, provides Adderall to low-income children in Cherokee County, north of Atlanta, to help them do better in school. Anderson told the *Times*, "I don't have a whole lot of choice. We've decided as a society that it's too expensive to modify the kid's environment. So we have to modify the kid."

Adderall is an amphetamine used to treat attention deficit hyperactivity disorder (ADHD). However, as the *Times* article suggests, pediatricians and pediatric psychiatrists have observed the growing practice of prescribing Adderall and other psychotropic drugs to enhance school performance in children who do not carry a diagnosis of ADHD. Essentially, bad school grades have become a treatable disease for doctors. As Anderson said of his prescribing, "People who are getting A's and B's, I won't give it to them."

The practice of physicians "medicalizing," or creating a disease out of disapproved behavior, has a long history. The ancient Greeks believed women exhibited specific emotional disorders that originated in the womb. For centuries the medical community was complicit in preventing women from assuming their full role in society by diagnosing them with "hysteria" (from the Greek for "uterus").

In the antebellum South, slaves who ran away from their masters were often diagnosed with "drapetomania," a "disease" that caused them to run away. Until 1973 the American Psychiatric Association classified homosexuality as a mental disorder. In defense of Anderson, his motives, while not defensible, are understandable. He and others are frustrated by low-income students trapped in failing schools and by the perceived societal neglect of those students' social and emotional needs.

Other trends also are at work here. Drugs are a lucrative shortcut. Performance-enhancing drugs in sports are ubiquitous (see Armstrong, Lance). Pharmaceutical companies seek to expand the indications for the use of their drugs ("off-labeling") to increase their profits. They pressure patients and doctors with aggressive marketing. Some physicians feel they have no option but to respond with the most accessible weapon at their disposal—the prescription pad.

Make no mistake, however; the attempt to improve healthy students' grades with Adderall, a practice fraught with danger, should be unequivocally condemned. Adderall is reasonably safe in the short-term treatment of

ADHD, but it can have serious and occasionally life-threatening neurologic and cardiovascular side effects. In addition the effects of Adderall on the developing central nervous system and the consequences of long-term use are poorly understood. Widespread prescription of the drug, especially when there is no known "correct" dose for poor school performance, would inevitably result in healthy children experiencing devastating side effects. The nature of Adderall as a stimulant also creates the potential in users for abuse and addiction; it is a widely sought drug on the black market.

An even more important consideration is whether Adderall actually works to improve grades in children without ADHD. The supposed benefits of Adderall as a study aid in healthy children are largely anecdotal. The causes of poor school performance are multifactorial, and many of those factors are not amenable to Adderall. Prescribing the drug without addressing basic remediable factors, such as parental involvement and improving nutrition, sleep habits, and physical fitness, borders on malpractice.

It would be disingenuous not to acknowledge that some students might benefit from Adderall. Its mechanism in ADHD is unknown, but its effect cannot be ignored. This is where science comes in. Today the trend in medicine is toward minimizing reliance on anecdotal experience and using instead evidence-based practice, studies to determine the safety and effectiveness of medications in selected populations.

If we seriously want to consider the use of Adderall to improve student performance, the government and the pharmaceutical companies should undertake well-designed, large-scale studies with appropriate informed consent for the children involved. This is the best way to maximize the benefit and minimize the harm—and even this is not perfect. Critics might reasonably object to the mind-control aspects of such studies. An understandable concern, but consider the alternative: doctors blindly prescribing these drugs and parents seeking them out for their children on an ad hoc basis.

In 1931 the English writer Aldous Huxley anticipated the Adderall issue in his novel *Brave New World*, the story of a futuristic society. One feature of that fictional society was the widespread use of a state-sponsored drug called "soma" (not to be confused with the real-life muscle relaxant of the same name). The literary soma was given to citizens to abolish feelings of unhappiness, anxiety, and rage, which had the associated effect of discouraging independent thought. In the story, Huxley described a solidarity service, a meeting where mindless conformity was encouraged through the administration of soma. "By the time the soma had begun to work, eyes shone, cheeks were flushed, the near light of universal benevolence broke out on every face in happy friendly smiles," Huxley wrote.

Huxley's brave new world was intended to be a dystopian nightmare. Does the widespread prescribing of Adderall pose a danger of creating a similar but real nightmare?

40

IS "LOW T" AN ACTUAL DISEASE?

The difficulty of defining disease is implied in the very structure
of the word: "dis-ease." So many different kinds of disturbances can
make a person feel not at ease and lead him to seek the aid
of a physician that the word ought to encompass most of the
difficulties inherent in the human condition.

—RENÉ JULES DUBOS

THE FOOD AND DRUG ADMINISTRATION (FDA) prides itself on taking
an active role in protecting consumers from the risks associated with
direct-to-consumer testing. Yet the FDA has been notably restrained on
the pharmaceutical marketing saturating the media and Internet concerning "low T," a condition that might be a "disease" or simply just a slick
advertising strategy to generate drugs sales.

Low T is the term for the decreasing blood level of the male hormone
testosterone in most men over the age of thirty. While extreme testosterone
deficiency is an actual inherited or acquired hormonal disease in a small
number of men, a gradual drop in testosterone occurs in normal aging

159

men (in contrast to the precipitous drop in sex hormones experienced by women at menopause). Although low T is a campaign to diagnose patients with "below normal" values of testosterone, this is problematic because the "normal" range for testosterone in the blood for males varies widely from age thirty through eighty. The ostensible purpose of diagnosing low T appears to be to create a market to sell testosterone supplements to a significant segment of middle-aged American and Canadian men. And it's working—in both countries testosterone use has increased exponentially in the past decade.

In a 2012 *Colbert Report,* Stephen Colbert facetiously, but accurately, described the billion-dollar industry: "A man on TV is selling me a miracle cure that will keep me young forever . . . for treating something called Low T, a pharmaceutical company–recognized condition affecting millions of men with low testosterone, previously known as getting older."

The pharmaceutical marketing of testosterone supplements avoids the scrutiny of the FDA by exploiting loopholes in the advertising laws. The FDA closely monitors prescription medication advertising—witness the fast-talking fine-print patter on television—but a company can circumvent that by creating a "disease-awareness" campaign. Low T advertising becomes part of disease awareness or in the industry jargon, having men take a proactive approach to their overall health. Commercials advise men to see their doctor for a checkup and to get tested for blood pressure, cholesterol—and testosterone. The unstated message being that low T is now a risk factor comparable to high blood pressure or elevated cholesterol.

That's what is meant by disease awareness. Of course a disease usually has symptoms, especially if a specific treatment is being marketed to the public. So according to the advertising, symptoms of low T include occasional fatigue, weight gain, mood swings, and decreased sex drive. Basically, symptoms endemic in aging baby-boomer males. In this way, low T is essentially transformed into a "quality of life" disease.

None of this means that testosterone supplements in patients with low testosterone levels have no benefit; testimonials to its effectiveness are not hard to come by. But testimonials are not the same as a proven scientific benefit; there is simply insufficient clinical literature on that count. A review article in *JAMA: The Journal of the American Medical Association* said, "Testosterone therapy results in only small improvements in lean body mass and body fat, libido, and sexual satisfaction, and has inconsistent (or no) effect on weight, depression, and lower extremity strength. Whether these effects are big enough to matter to patients is unknown."

At the same time, there is no guarantee that treating low T is completely safe. Some cardiologists worry that one important side effect of testosterone supplementation may be accelerated coronary heart disease. As with the benefits of testosterone supplementation, the risks have not received enough scientific scrutiny to date. Since the low T advertisements are careful not to refer to any specific medicine, there is no obligation to mention any downsides to treatment, unlike warnings that must be included for prescription drug advertising.

Today middle-aged men find themselves in a similar position to women of a generation ago. Then, the medical community pushed for estrogen and progestin supplementation in women during and after menopause on the theory that hormone supplementation would confer protection against heart disease. It was not until 2002 that a Women's Health Initiative long-term study of hormone replacement in 160,000 women failed to demonstrate such protection. In fact it was suggested the treatment might have increased the danger of heart disease and cancer.

If there is a difference between then and now, it is that the pharmaceutical industry has wholeheartedly embraced the modern direct-to-consumer marketing approach that bypasses the physician. While there are undeniably public health benefits to the direct-to-consumer approach in terms of promoting health awareness, there is a fine line between that and a manufactured campaign for a pseudodisease. And as the case of low T illustrates, there is a lot of money to be made straddling that line. That straddle may not be illegal or even unethical. But it's close, and until greater study is done on the risks and benefits of testosterone supplementation in low T, the FDA should pay special attention to this new disease.

41

JUST BECAUSE YOU ARE RICH DOESN'T MEAN YOU ARE SMART

---

*I'll get killed for saying this but I'm not so against steroids
if they're administered under proper supervision
and there is no long-term damage.*

—MARK CUBAN

A T A SPEECH at the University of Pittsburgh, Mark Cuban, the Dallas Mavericks' billionaire owner, gave his opinion on steroids and sports by noting that medical practices like LASIK eye surgery and Tommy John surgery already improve athletic performance. He asked if that's not considered cheating, why the double standard when it comes to drugs? "You administer them properly and fairly and set the rules strictly, as long as in doing so we recognize there are no negative long-term health-impact issues."

Cuban, a superrich windbag who lacks a mind-mouth filter, gets more publicity than he deserves. His uninformed pronouncements reflect the sentiment that steroids should be made available to any professional or amateur adult athlete who wants them. And he has support from some experts who claim the harm in steroids is minimal and represents nothing more than a technology advance, no different from fiberglass vaulting poles or specially designed swimsuits.

In analyzing the issue, medical ethicist Norman Fost cited Ben Johnson in the 1988 Olympics, vilified for using performance-enhancing drugs while American swimmer Janet Evans was hailed for winning a gold medal when she wore a top-secret, high-tech fabric swimsuit. The argument is basically the harm of these drugs is overblown and most side effects are either short term or merely cosmetic. The unfair advantage the drugs confer would be minimized if everyone had access to these drugs.

Yet the short-term physical and psychological side effects have been well documented, even if they are occasionally overstated. As for long-term effects, nobody knows since there has never been any long-term evaluation. It took nearly two decades for the incredible performances of East German female swimmers to come under scrutiny. Because so much is unknown, these drugs must be considered far riskier than LASIK or Tommy John surgery. The athlete who accepts the unknown risks will always have an advantage over those who prefer "to play clean." But there is no basis to compare these drugs to equipment advances like high-tech swimsuits that confer advantage but do not jeopardize athletes' health.

The most compelling argument is the danger these drugs pose to children. Professional athletes' success with performance-enhancing drugs is a main reason the drugs are sought by teenagers—and a strong argument for banning them at the professional level. Even Norman Fost acknowledges the risks to young people. He favors testing young athletes. His punishment for those distributing drugs to them is simple and straightforward—"Hanging followed by a fair trial."

There is no bright line between seeking a competitive edge and "cheating." But there is such a thing as cheating. Competitive sports are inherently difficult. Even the greatest competitors are humbled by their sport's limitations. Mark Buerhle, untainted by any drug allegations, pitched a perfect game for the White Sox in 2009 and set a major league record by retiring forty-five consecutive batters. Right after that he failed to win a game for six weeks. Even in his prime, Tiger Woods occasionally failed to make a tournament cut.

Performance-enhancing drugs permit athletes to circumvent the natural limitations of their sport. The drugs confer an unfair advantage, even if unproven scientifically. Athletes using these compounds cheat their fellow competitors and cheat their sport. Many athletes elect not to use performance-enhancing drugs but are reluctant to point out a problem they know exists. This "conspiracy of silence" extends to coaches and others (especially the Major League Baseball Players' Union), creating a public crisis of confidence in sports. In the case of complicit sports physicians, it's a clear dereliction of duty.

If today's situation is disturbing, genetic engineering advances may soon permit scientists to inject genes into target muscles and exponentially increase performance. Gene transfer therapy, already theoretically possible, might allow the body to repair and re-create damaged tissue immediately. Such techniques might be undetectable by testing. Competitive athletics could become caricatured entertainment—sluggers hitting 250 home runs per season, pitchers with 115 mph fastballs, and sprinters running 100 meters in 7 seconds.

The future is problematic for the sports culture and society at large. Performance-enhancing drugs mean greater paychecks for athletes and billionaire owners like Mark Cuban. But they tarnish competition and endanger the lives of athletes and would-be athletes. Mark Cuban's foolish belief is that he can extract the value from performance-enhancing drugs without realizing the eventual cost.

42

FLYING TOO CLOSE TO THE SUN

Don't decide on a dog based on looks, much like with people,
looks and first impressions can be deceiving.

—Elizabeth Holmes, founder and CEO of Theranos

I N 2004 ELIZABETH HOLMES, a nineteen-year-old Stanford dropout, created Theranos, a health care start-up that was once valued as high as $9 billion, which gave her a one-time net worth north of $4 billion. *Forbes* described her as "the youngest self-made female billionaire in the world." Like other Silicon Valley wunderkind, she was instantly hailed as a genius and transformed into a media darling, her every trivial observation, even about dogs, regarded as wisdom worthy of Confucius.

Unfortunately, a federal investigation of Theranos showed Ms. Holmes that in the matter of looks and first impressions, some witty quotes can be like some dogs—they can deceive, then turn around and bite.

Theranos was developed based on its "breakthrough technology"; the company claimed it could run dozens of blood tests from a fingerstick instead of a sample drawn from a vein. Anyone who has ever experienced difficulty having his or her blood drawn would appreciate the less cumbersome fingerstick approach. In addition Theranos advertised it could make its results available at a far lower price than other laboratories.

The reason blood drawn from a vein has traditionally been used for testing is because the consistent mixing of blood in veins yields dependable sample results; a fingerstick blood sample is not as uniform. Blood from tiny vessels also contains fluid from tissues where the stick is performed. This is not a problem with small molecules like glucose, where fingerstick samples are reliable—that is what home glucose kits do. But the mixture of tissue fluid and blood changes the concentration of larger molecules like proteins and cholesterol, so fingerstick results are less consistent than that of blood from veins. Theranos claimed to have solved this problem with its proprietary laboratory technology.

At the inception, Ms. Holmes did a brilliant job of promoting the mystique of Theranos. In the name of empowering patients, she touted her company's mission to permit consumers to monitor their own health with inexpensive and easy-to-run blood tests. Theranos's original board of directors was a "who's who" of people like Henry Kissinger and George Schultz—long on business and government clout but suspiciously short on experience in chemistry, pathology, and laboratory testing.

With one notable exception, business journalists were charmed by Ms. Holmes's marketing approach, as were venture capital firms and other Silicon Valley business moguls. She was compared to Steve Jobs. Soon respected health care companies like the Cleveland Clinic and Walgreens cut deals to partner with Theranos, and this only increased the company's cachet.

But there was always a sticking point, no pun intended. Because Theranos operated in secrecy, it refused to divulge its methodology or allow its laboratory results to be widely tested against industry standards. The *Wall Street Journal*, the exception among business publications, raised serious doubts about the Theranos technology, the reliability of their test results, and the lack of medical experience of its board of directors.

The company came under scrutiny by the Centers for Medicare and Medicaid Services, which examined whether the Theranos technology actually works. Theranos admitted that thousands of its laboratory tests from 2014 and 2015 were invalid. Other investigations probed the possibility that Theranos misled investors. The company's chief operating officer was forced to retire, and to assuage the business community, Ms. Holmes reconstituted the entire Theranos board by adding experienced medical and laboratory experts. After a flurry of lawsuits and settlements, Theranos has burned through large amounts of cash and may have difficulty raising more in the future. Walgreens has terminated its partnership with the company.

At Stanford, when Ms. Holmes first came up with the idea for a cheap, rapid fingerstick approach to blood testing, she decided on the company name Theranos as a combination of two words with ancient Greek derivation, *therapy* and *diagnosis*. Perhaps her appreciation for the ancient Greeks did not extend to the myth of Daedalus and his son, Icarus. Daedalus was an inventor and innovator, the kind Ms. Holmes aspired to be. Trapped on an island, Daedalus, undaunted that man had never left the ground before, invented wings made of wax so that he and Icarus could escape by flying away. Despite his father's warnings, Icarus, enamored of his newfound ability, flew too close to the sun, causing the wax to melt, and he crashed into the sea.

Lessons for young Silicon Valley entrepreneurs: a little more study of Greek mythology never hurts. The promise of a "breakthrough technology" cost Daedalus his most precious possession, and flying too close to the sun can be dangerous.

43

HOW MOVIES AND PHARMACEUTICALS ARE ALIKE

Everything I learned I learned from the movies.

—AUDREY HEPBURN

WHILE YOU'RE BUSY filling your tank with $2.50 a gallon gasoline, you may not have noticed the price of some other commodities—movies (average ticket $8–$10) and medicine (50 percent rise in the past fifteen years)—has risen far faster than that of gasoline in the past four decades. The honchos running Hollywood and the pharmaceutical companies must marvel at their good fortune when the public expends its venom at big oil. Cruising under the radar, hands in our wallets, the studio and pharmaceutical executives could lunch together and exchange tips on business strategies and problems their industries share:

1. *Both industries count on blockbusters.* Movie studios constantly seek the next *Titanic* (total gross—$2 billion), while drug companies look for the next Humira (2014 sales—$11.8 billion). The phenomenal success of

early blockbusters decades ago—*Jaws* in the theater, Zantac in the drug store—reconfigured both industries. Blockbusters reduced the pressure to turn out a steady number of good products with modest sales. By the same token, art house films and orphan drugs produced by smaller independents, which show meager returns on investment, are tolerated grudgingly, if at all.

2. *The safest financial bets are sequels.* By barraging the public with countless sequels and remakes, Hollywood displays its lack of creativity—consider *Pirates of the Caribbean* and *The Fast and the Furious*. Likewise, a pharmaceutical industry staple are "me-too" drugs; witness the profusion of cholesterol-lowering medicines. If drugs were movies, Crestor would be Mevacor II. As with sequels, the "me-too" drug strategy replaces an emphasis on creativity with reaping profits from known commodities. Good science becomes less important than good marketing.

3. *Costs and uncertainties of movie and drug development mean both industries must realize large returns quickly to offset expected failures along the way.* Movie revenue occurs primarily in the first year of release. The most desirable movie, the one most likely to recoup costs, is one that can be franchised and incorporated into toys, games, and theme parks. Drugs take a long time to develop and generate revenue for a longer period, but the motivation is similar—when the patent expires, the generic pill sells for twenty-five cents. (Patents extend out twenty years and are necessary to protect investment but essentially act as a short-term monopoly.) The pharmaceutical equivalent of the theme park is the nongeneric drug you must take for the rest of your life.

4. *Success is tied to marketing and distribution costs.* Technology, including computers and genomics, has brought down the cost of producing movies and drugs, respectively. But the costs of advertising and distribution (and in the case of drugs, Food and Drug Administration approval) continue to increase. Consequently, in both industries, small independent producers (and for pharmaceuticals, universities and the government) now do much of the exciting new work. Industry giants sometimes function as

distribution companies, buying their new products from small producers by promising the necessary promotion in exchange for a share of profits.

5. *Companies can get too big and too cautious.* They lose their tolerance for risk while their size allows them to accept costly failures. Occasionally, mergers or acquisitions of smaller companies with good products can lead to an unhealthy concentration of power in a small number of major studios and drug firms in the United States. The new, larger conglomerate is often less responsive to the public, and product innovation suffers. As past mergers in both sectors demonstrate, sometimes 1 + 1 = 1.5.

6. *Both industries confront serious threats in the courtroom.* Hollywood fights desperately to control online piracy and new technologies that facilitate copying and sharing films. The pharmaceutical giants, always mindful of patent infringement, always face the danger of mass tort litigation. Companies forced to "lawyer up" pass on their legal fees as an increasing part of the cost of that movie ticket or bottle of medicine.

7. *Accounting practices remain mysterious.* When the late columnist Art Buchwald successfully sued Paramount for stealing his idea for the movie *Coming to America*, Paramount claimed, straight-faced, they lost money on one of the highest-grossing movies of all time (a settlement was later reached). Meanwhile, court rulings that most pricing information is proprietary and companies shouldn't have to open their books have protected the pharmaceutical industry for years.

Today both industries thrive because the public loves movies and depends on medicine. They may pick our pockets, but we need them. The final similarity? Some of what they sell us is a waste of time and money. The really good stuff can change or save our lives, but the really bad stuff is sometimes deadly or just deadly dull.

44

UNPROFESSIONAL
PROFESSIONALS

A good reputation is more valuable than money.

—PUBLILIUS SYRUS

MANY PHYSICIANS THESE DAYS are seeing their incomes squeezed as hospitals buy their practices and insurance companies and the government come down hard on reimbursements. One recourse for this loss of income is for physicians to augment their incomes through expert testimony in the courtroom. By itself there is nothing wrong with this; the system certainly needs more independent experts willing to explain medical science to the lay public. The key word is *independent.*

Unfortunately, the money to be made can prompt some physicians to advocate too strongly for one side or the other by offering opinions that stretch the limits of advocacy. From there it is only a short journey to junk science. And even courts have trouble identifying junk science; there are different standards in different jurisdictions.

Throw in to this mix the fact that both plaintiff and defense lawyers are always on the lookout for doctors with favorable bias toward their sides. To build their legal cases, this is often much more important to the lawyers than the search for "the truth." In medical litigation it is a common practice for lawyers to keep rolodexes of expert physicians categorized as "pro-defense" or "pro-plaintiff." This is a tacit dismissal of the possibility of the unbiased expert. One of the first questions physicians are always asked at an expert deposition is how often they work for the defense versus how often they work for plaintiffs. This standard question is done to establish that "pro-defense" versus "pro-plaintiff" classification. Time was when if a physician testified for only one side, it was tacitly assumed he or she was biased. Lawyers have countered that assumption with the argument that if someone is a renowned expert in a specific area, say blood clots in the lung, who better to testify that the diagnosis was missed than this expert? Hence 95 percent of the time that expert testifies the blood clot was missed. No bias, just expertise.

There is no simple solution to this problem of the search for the unbiased expert. Most experienced attorneys understand this and adapt appropriately. The amount of money tied up in medical litigation is so great that conflicts of interest and unscrupulous advocacy will always be a point of contention. The answer does not lie, as some physicians propose, in eliminating lay juries from the equation. Whatever the flaws in how it judges cases, the lay public must remain a part of the system even if it means an occasional outrageous settlement or unjust jury verdict.

Years ago I served as an expert witness in several cases. I split my time almost equally between plaintiff and defense, and I accepted only cases I thought had merit, one way or another. I faced a number of formidable experts on the other side, some of whom I felt were scrupulously honest, others who I felt were not. Doing this, I learned a valuable lesson. The primary purpose of medical litigation (and much other litigation) is not to establish "the truth"; to assure good medicine is practiced; or even to dispense justice, whatever your concept of justice is. The purpose of medical litigation is to resolve disputes, when one party says X and another party says Y. (Consider it a civilized advance from the time our long-ago ancestors settled disputes by means of violence.) This doesn't mean that better medicine doesn't result from medical litigation—it often does. And in many cases, the truth is established and justice is realized. But those are the by-products of a dispute resolution system that is admittedly imperfect but may be the best we can do.

The best approach to minimizing outrageous advocacy and junk science is greater scrutiny by the professional societies, medical and legal, that oversee their members' behavior. But unless and until the professional societies are willing to publicly condemn unscrupulous and avaricious behavior, the rest of us will be at the mercy of the occasional unprofessional professional.

45

ASSISTED SUICIDE: HOW CAN WE BE SURE WHEN IT IS RIGHT?

When life and death are at stake,
rules and obligations go by the board.

—ALBERT EINSTEIN

BEFORE HIS DEATH IN 2011, Dr. Jack Kevorkian was released from prison after serving seven years of a ten- to twenty-five-year sentence for the 1998 second-degree murder/mercy killing of Thomas Youk, who suffered from Lou Gehrig's disease. Kevorkian looked none the worse for wear as he relentlessly made the talk show rounds on the *Today Show, Good Morning, America, Larry King*, and on *60 Minutes* with Mike Wallace. The *60 Minutes* appearance represented a comeback of sorts since it was the *60 Minutes* story on the administration of lethal drugs to Youk that led to Kevorkian's original conviction.

According to his lawyer, Kevorkian was offered speaking fees of $50–$100,000 to discuss his experience and advocacy for assisted suicide. But while Kevorkian became a media celebrity and brought renewed attention to the subject, an ominous development on assisted suicide in Europe has escaped notice in the United States.

In Switzerland an inconspicuous medical clinic known as Dignitas is located among a block of studio apartments in a modest suburb of Zurich. Founded in 1998 by a Swiss human rights lawyer, Dignitas was created to take advantage of Switzerland's liberal assisted suicide laws. A patient can become a member of Dignitas and apply in writing for assisted suicide with a doctor's note certifying illness, prognosis, and pain. The clinic's volunteer staff certifies the information and provides the patient with a lethal cocktail of barbiturates, which the patient then self-administers. Dignitas has helped over two thousand patients die in Switzerland.

Dignitas has become the focal point of a "death tourism" industry for citizens of other European Union countries who travel to Switzerland to end their lives discreetly in one of the suburban studio flats. Germans and Britons are the main travelers, and over three hundred patients from Great Britain have died in the Swiss clinic. But now questions are emerging as to whether some foreign clients who were helped to die were simply depressed rather than terminally ill or in incurable pain. It appears some of these clients may have been given lethal cocktails without appropriate investigation into their medical conditions.

The London *Daily Telegraph* reported that a German woman who died in the Dignitas clinic presented the staff with phony papers stating she was suffering from terminal liver cirrhosis. It was later discovered she was suffering from depression and alcoholism. Other death tourists may have also provided spurious medical and psychiatric records, which the staff failed to verify. A member of the Swiss regulatory agency on biomedical ethics admitted, "We suspect there could have been cases where people who suffered from a temporary depression have been helped to their deaths."

Here in the United States, observers relooked at the 130 patients Dr. Kevorkian admitted to helping commit suicide, some of whom traveled great distances to avail themselves of his services. Several of these patients did not have terminal illnesses, and although many suffered from chronic conditions such as multiple sclerosis, at least a few did not have any life-threatening condition at autopsy, a fact lost in the media attention at the time.

If his interviews were any indication, Jack Kevorkian did not mellow after his prison stint. He was a well-read, clever man who lacked introspection. He readily stated that physicians who engage in assisted suicide must be free of conflicts of interest, and he admitted that he never accepted money for his services. But he never acknowledged a different form of conflict of interest. Before his first assisted suicide, he was an obscure retired pathologist. Then his exploits brought him unimaginable fame—media attention and national celebrity that he enjoyed again after his release from prison. In his defense the lure of all those television cameras would be hard for anyone to resist. But that level of fame, a conflict of interest no different than taking money, may have caused him to cut corners even by his own iconoclastic standards.

In his 1991 book, *Prescription Medicide: The Goodness of Planned Death*, Kevorkian extolled the virtues of assisted suicide while never acknowledging its limitations. He wrote, "Reverence for the traditional Hippocratic basis of medical practice is vacuous nostalgia, childish daydreaming."

The question of physician-assisted suicide has never been as cut and dried as Kevorkian portrayed it. When rules and obligations go by the board, as they may have in Switzerland, doctors are left with the moral dilemma Kevorkian seemed oblivious to: When we take another's life, how can we ever be sure what we are doing is right?

V

THE BRAVE NEW WORLD
OF NEUROLOGY

46

BETTER USE OF OUR NEW TOOLS FOR PATIENTS IN COMA

And men should know that from nothing else but from the brain
came joys, delights, laughter and jests, and sorrows, griefs,
despondency and lamentations. And by this, in an especial manner,
we acquire wisdom and knowledge, and see and hear
and know what are foul, and what are fair,
what sweet and what unsavory.

—HIPPOCRATES

I TREATED PATIENTS IN INTENSIVE CARE UNITS all over the country for forty years, and patients in coma were unquestionably the most emotionally wrenching group to care for. Often the reason for coma was tragic, sudden, and unexpected. A family would come to the hospital in stunned silence and see their loved one, who had been alert and awake hours before, now lying in a hospital bed, unresponsive from trauma, stroke, cardiac arrest, or drug overdose.

Eventually all families asked the same two questions: first, what happened to their loved one, then invariably, "Will he (or she) wake up?" And because some uncertainty was always present, I usually answered, "I'm not sure." Depending on the cause, some patients ultimately woke up and others didn't, but in some cases, the uncertainty over whether the patient would recover might last days, weeks, or even months.

In patients with brain injuries from various causes, the extent of damage and the level of consciousness ("Doctor, can my father hear us talking?") has always been difficult to judge. Hence the ability to predict which patients would recover from coma has, of necessity, been imprecise. This is primarily because most physician judgment has traditionally been based on bedside clinical examination of the patient. Although clinical examination is essential to a good evaluation, it is limited in the ability to ascertain which patients will wake up. A significant fraction of patients are misdiagnosed when clinical examination is used without other tests.

In the 1980s, the CT scan became a widespread adjunct to physical examination and has helped immeasurably, primarily when the cause of coma is not obvious. But the CT scan is essentially an anatomic tool— that is, it shows normal and abnormal brain structures but does not tell us about brain function and is not an especially good predictive tool for patients in coma.

Likewise, the MRI, introduced two decades after the CT, represented an advance in the care of coma patients. The MRI is often more precise than the CT scan, and it can show blood flow to the brain and how the brain uses oxygen. But even with the MRI, the uncertainty associated with recovery from coma is substantial. We still do not know exactly who will wake up and who will remain comatose.

A study by Belgian researchers in the journal *Current Biology* suggests that a newer brain-imaging technique known as positron emission tomography (the PET scan) provides a strong suggestion of which comatose patients are likely to recover consciousness. Unlike CT, the PET scan is an indicator of brain metabolism and shows how the brain uses glucose.

While not perfect, the PET scan appears to be better in quantifying brain activity and predicting recovery in comatose patients than clinical examination. Future studies are likely to show that a combination of imaging tests, combined with good examination of the patient, will be superior to any one of them alone.

Only recently has the PET scan been used to test diagnostic accuracy in actual patients. Until now it has been primarily a research tool, and doctors have been reluctant, perhaps too reluctant, to use it in everyday patient care because of the expense and unfamiliarity with the new technology.

Commenting on a 2014 study in the *Lancet*, two prominent neuroscientists suggested the use of PET scans in brain-injured patients should become common. They predicted that the PET scan will revolutionize neurology: "Functional brain imaging is expensive and technically challenging, but it will almost certainly become cheaper and easier. In the future, we will probably look back in amazement at how we were ever able to practice without it."

The brain is a remarkable organ; over twenty-five hundred years ago, Greek physicians understood it to be the seat of consciousness. And yet today, centuries later, our understanding of the brain remains in its infancy. The incidence of brain injury continues to increase, and at a cost of billions of dollars annually, we remain challenged to predict which patients will recover. These amazing new tools may help us successfully confront the challenge of patients in coma.

47

HOW A TELLTALE HEART COULD CHANGE MEDICINE FOREVER

I say, there came to my ears a low, dull, quick sound,
such as a watch makes when enveloped in cotton. I knew that
sound well too. It was the beating of the old man's heart.

—EDGAR ALLAN POE, "THE TELL-TALE HEART"

"THE TELL-TALE HEART" is a chilling 1843 short story by Edgar
Allan Poe about a man whose disturbed conscience is haunted by
the sound of a heart that will not stop beating. The real-life telltale heart
is the tragic story of seventeen-year-old Jahi McMath, who was diagnosed
as "brain dead" over three years ago but whose heart still beats. The case
generated a lawsuit that could overturn a half century of established belief
and haunt the conscience of medicine.

McMath's heart and blood pressure have been stable for more than
three and a half years, an unanticipated finding extremely rare with the
diagnosis of brain death. Perhaps in her case, the original diagnosis was

wrong, a disturbing possibility, or more likely it simply means we must rethink the twentieth-century concept of brain death.

In December 2013, following a routine tonsillectomy for sleep apnea, McMath suffered a cardiac arrest and massive brain damage from lack of oxygen to the brain. Several neurologists found she demonstrated no sign of cerebral electrical activity, no blood flow to her brain, and could not breathe on her own. She was diagnosed as "brain dead"; a California coroner issued a death certificate, and the hospital prepared to discontinue her ventilator.

In a legal proceeding independent from the current lawsuit, McMath's family went to court in 2014 to prevent her from being removed from the ventilator. The judge assigned an expert from Stanford to examine McMath, and he concurred with the diagnosis of brain death. Technically McMath, brain dead, was no longer a living person.

Despite this, her family subsequently received court approval and removed her from the hospital to a facility willing to care for her. She is currently on a ventilator, being fed through a feeding tube. Her heart has been beating far longer than that of nearly any other brain-dead patient, a troublesome fact most experts have failed to acknowledge since the first court hearing. When McMath's family initially went to court, most bioethicists and doctors familiar with brain death felt the family's interests, while understandable, should not supersede the law. The conventional thinking was that the judge's decision to keep McMath on a ventilator was in error; once McMath was declared legally dead, the court should have ordered the ventilator disconnected. Without the ventilator to breathe for her, her heart certainly would have stopped in minutes.

The possibility remains, however small, that experts may have been wrong, and a medical malpractice lawsuit may force reconsideration of the issue of whether McMath is alive or dead. Here's why: in cases of properly diagnosed brain death, no patient has ever recovered to come off a ventilator. The only things keeping the heart beating are the ventilator and occasionally drugs given to sustain the blood pressure, usually given when the patient is an organ donor. However, even in brain death, machines and drugs are usually not enough to sustain the heart. Even with the patient connected to the ventilator, the heart will usually stop fairly soon. Within a few hours to a few days, patients "die" in the widely understood sense. There have been isolated cases of pregnant women who were brain dead but kept on life support until their babies were delivered. Outside of those, there are only a handful of reports of brain-dead patients on ventilators whose hearts beat for more than three months, and in some of those cases, the correct diagnosis of brain death has been questioned.

Because McMath's heart has continued to beat far longer, the new lawsuit against the hospital and doctors who originally performed the surgery reopens an area of life and death once thought settled. In California, damages are legally capped for the wrongful death of a child, but there is no cap, and damages could run into tens of millions of dollars, if the child is injured but still alive, as the suit claims. So the court might actually have to revisit the question, "Is Jahi McMath alive or dead?"

Unlike the cases of Terri Schiavo and Karen Ann Quinlan, who were not brain dead and could breathe without ventilator assistance, the issue in McMath's case is not whether she will ever regain consciousness. That would be completely out of the realm of experience. The question is the meaning of brain death as death of a person and whether traditional diagnostic criteria require reexamination in view of McMath's unusual situation. The answers are essential to neurology, organ transplantation, and public policy.

In 1968 the medical community outlined specific neurologic tests that, if fulfilled, indicated a person was brain dead. This created an alternative definition of death, which has been accepted legally in every state. Since then a number of new diagnostic tests, including PET scans and MRIs, have been developed that measure brain activity more precisely. With such an important medicolegal issue at stake and with the older criteria likely to be questioned in McMath's case, these new tests, while not used routinely in the diagnosis of brain death, may have an important future role.

The question of the exact moment life ends is conceptual—it can never be conclusively settled. Albert Einstein once observed that a single experiment could prove his most elaborate theory wrong. Likewise, the sad case of young Jahi McMath and her "telltale heart" have the potential to change the medical community's understanding of brain death.

48

THE NEW PARADIGM OF
ASSISTIVE TECHNOLOGY

Any sufficiently advanced technology is indistinguishable from magic.
—ARTHUR C. CLARKE

WHEN HE WAS IN HIS EARLY THIRTIES, former National Football League (NFL) player Steve Gleason contracted amyotrophic lateral sclerosis (ALS), a motor neuron disease that robs people of muscle control and currently affects about twenty thousand Americans. As the disease progresses, it eventually leaves patients paralyzed but spares their eye movements and leaves their minds intact.

Because patients with advanced ALS cannot talk, they need help communicating, and Gleason, confined to a wheelchair, has been working with Microsoft to develop "assistive technology": new tablet computers that use eye-tracking technology and speech-generating software. Gleason has described his personal progress, "I can do anything an ordinary person can do on a tablet computer—talk, videoconference, text, stream music, buy

Christmas presents online, pay bills, tweet." He and Microsoft are currently working on a wheelchair he can drive with his eyes. What they are doing was unimaginable a generation ago.

As Microsoft demonstrates with Steve Gleason, this is a chance for the Silicon Valley companies like Apple and Google to develop research capabilities and customized products for the health care market. But it doesn't even take a giant like Microsoft to create revolutionary assistive technology. Through crowdsourcing, a small Israeli company is currently developing an affordable prototype device for patients with locked-in syndrome, a type of brain damage that resembles ALS. The device, an infrared camera connected to a pair of glasses, records the user's eye movements and communicates them to an attached microcomputer. The computer translates those eye movements into programmed commands, which can then be transmitted via headphones, speaker, or smartphone. Once, paralyzed patients with locked-in syndrome had no one to speak for them; now with the right training, they may soon be able to "speak" for themselves.

In rehabilitation medicine, the use of computers, tablets, and smartphones is only now emerging. As the American population ages, there are more people surviving with strokes, Parkinson's disease, multiple sclerosis, and other similar disorders who could participate in everyday activities by using these assistive technologies. This situation is not limited to the elderly; there are currently thousands of young patients with spinal cord trauma, brain trauma, or neuromuscular diseases who would likewise benefit from the latest hardware and software. For patients with neurologic diseases, vision problems, or other disabilities, these tools are essential to communicate or get around. In some cases, these devices may also be the patient's only means of interacting with others and combating loneliness.

These patients often need customized devices because standardized equipment may not be right—tablet screens are often too small, and patients may not have the dexterity or strength to use smartphone keys. However, it is not simply a matter of machinery. Just as important, these patients need a well-trained therapist to help them since they may not have the experience with new technology or may be unaware of what the technology can actually do. Hospitals currently employ specially trained therapists to help people move (physical therapy), to aid people with breathing problems (respiratory therapy), help those with difficulty communicating (speech therapy), and return people to daily activity (occupational therapy). But with the advent of new, customized devices, there is a need for specialized therapists whose primary focus is to evaluate the specific assistive technology needs of patients with disabilities and help them use personalized technology. With the exception of a limited number of specialty facilities, few hospitals have such a therapist.

Especially for tech-savvy young people, all this could present a genuine opportunity for a prospective start-up career—assistive technology therapy. The call should go out to hospitals and universities to devise curricula and work with other therapists, teaching prospective assistive technology therapists about different conditions and the specific limitations those conditions present for patients, as well as the solutions available through emerging technology. Assistive technology therapists could then become part of every hospital, large clinic, rehabilitation center, and nursing home. Imagine a cadre of trained professionals working with disabled patients, custom-fitting them for the right device, and helping them learn (or relearn) not just how to communicate and move about but how to search the Internet, use social media, and even play video games.

Medicine's early adaptation to the computer age was to develop devices like the electronic medical record, the computerized scanner, and the robot that can perform surgery. Although these innovations have been undeniable advances in patient care, they have all had the perverse effect of causing less interaction between caregivers and patients. The resident typing into the electronic record does not make eye contact with his patient; the consultant looking at the scan no longer performs a physical exam on her patient; the surgeon, once intimately involved, now operates with a robot at a distance from the patient.

But medicine can also use computer technology and still reverse this trend. In the future we need more assistive technology therapists, a critical first step to creating a new, personalized "high-tech, high-touch" approach. Combined with new devices and software, you will see miracles.

49

GOOGLE, GENE MAPPING, AND
A CHRISTMAS CAROL

Are these the shadows of the things that Will be,
or are they shadows of things that May be, only?

—Ebenezer Scrooge in Charles Dickens's *A Christmas Carol*

SERGEY BRIN, a forty-four-year-old Russian émigré, comes to work
in T-shirts, jeans, and sneakers. He revealed a secret about himself on
his personal blog that may be important to you. With slicked-back hair and
a fair complexion that make him look ten years younger, he could easily
be mistaken for your typical Starbucks trainee. But a quick Google search
identifies Sergey Brin as the fourth-youngest billionaire in the world and
fifth-richest man in the United States. That quick Google search increased
Brin's fortune since he happens to be a cofounder of Google Inc.

The secret Brin told the world was that he has a genetic mutation
that increases his chances of contracting Parkinson's disease later in life.
Parkinson's disease, a progressive degenerative central nervous system dis-

order, currently affects 1 percent of people over sixty-five. The mean age of onset is between fifty-five and sixty (some are stricken much earlier). As it progresses it causes tremors, and patients experience difficulty with everyday activities, including walking, speech, and swallowing. Mr. Brin's mother suffers from Parkinson's disease, as did his late aunt.

Until recently, Parkinson's was not thought to be heritable since there was no obvious pattern running in families. That thinking has been changed by genetic mapping, a technology that will soon be commonly available and inexpensive. Brin acknowledges that the implications of his results aren't yet clear because it's still uncertain which patients with the mutation will ultimately develop Parkinson's. Studies suggest having the mutation does confer a much-higher chance of developing Parkinson's for him than for the average person, though the exact probability is not known. In addition it is unknown whether the risk can be minimized or, alternatively, increased by cofactors such as diet, lifestyle, or environmental exposures.

The mutation was discovered when he took a mapping test of his DNA offered by a company called 23andME. (Coincidentally, 23andME was originally a partner to Google and was cofounded by Brin's wife. Silicon Valley legend is that Brin and his partner started Google in her sister's garage after leaving Stanford in the mid-1990s.) Brin said he didn't intend to have his DNA mapped to check for a Parkinson's risk but was glad to have the information.

Here's why his secret is important. Brin has taken a proactive approach to the news.

I know early in my life something I am substantially predisposed to. I now have the opportunity to adjust my life to reduce those odds. I also have the opportunity to perform and support research into this disease long before it may affect me. And, regardless of my own health it can help my family members as well as others. I feel fortunate to be in this position. Until the fountain of youth is discovered, all of us will have some conditions in our old age only we don't know what they will be. I have

a better guess than almost anyone else for what ills may be mine—and I
have decades to prepare for it.

Many people would, quite understandably, elect not to know they
carry the genes of a serious disease that may manifest itself in the future.
Yet Brin's revelation about his personal DNA is a watershed moment in
twenty-first-century medicine. With a personal fortune of billions of dollars,
Google's immense resources, and the support of the scientific community,
he can explore the frontiers of medical genetics, including how diseases
are expressed through genes, which patients will respond to specific medications or experience serious side effects, and whether there are ways to
prevent the diseases patients are predisposed to—in effect, how to change
their destiny.

Part of Sergey Brin's quest is to change his own destiny. It is a timeless
theme of literary and cinematic fiction. In classic Greek literature, Oedipus
Rex was told his future but still couldn't prevent his tragic fate. In contemporary fiction, heroes with extraordinary powers like Superman valiantly
attempt to alter the future to rescue people. Now in real life, scientists will
observe, and the rest of the world may benefit from Sergey Brin's case history to see whether genetic destiny can be modified.

The plight of the young billionaire with slicked-back hair recalls that
of a fictional wealthy man who was also shown a glimpse of his future,
Charles Dickens's elderly Ebenezer Scrooge. After Scrooge had his own
ignominious end revealed in *A Christmas Carol*, he vowed to change his
ways—and in doing so, he changed his future and that of those around
him. Scrooge presaged Brin's current efforts by musing, "Men's courses will
foreshadow certain ends, to which, if they persevered in, they must lead.
But if the courses be departed from, the ends will change."

50

I HAVE LOST MY MENTAL FACULTIES BUT AM QUITE WELL

Young men be not proud in the presence of a decaying old man; he was once that which you are, he is now that which you will be.

—POPE CLEMENT III

WHEN ROBERT BYRD was ninety-one years old, he had been a senator for fifty years and was fourth in line of presidential succession. At ninety-two, Sumner Redstone was the executive chairman of CBS and Viacom, two of the world's most powerful media companies. Fidel Castro, supreme leader of Cuba since the 1959 revolution, was a relative youngster when he died at ninety. No one in the inner circles of these three powerful men publicly questioned their mental capacity to do their jobs until near the end of their lives. Their aides would be understandably reluctant to openly utter the R word, perhaps fearing involuntary retirement themselves.

But when he was seventy-five, another US senator, Pete Domenici (R-NM), announced he would not seek a sixth Senate term, in part because of a debilitating central nervous system disease that commonly causes behavior disorders and dementia. By doing so, Domenici avoided the experience of the late Strom Thurmond (R-SC), the longest-serving senator in history when he retired in 2002 at age one hundred. During his last years, Thurmond chaired the Armed Services Committee amid rumors he wasn't always cognizant of the goings on around him. His final appearances consisted primarily of reading opening statements prepared by staff members, who nervously hovered close by.

This portends an impending societal dilemma: When people in positions of authority and responsibility can no longer function effectively, who will decide whether they should continue, and how? In the next three decades, several million Americans are projected to develop Alzheimer's disease and related degenerative neurologic conditions similar to that of Senator Domenici.

These neurologic diseases and the demographics of aging baby boomers present a huge problem for both the private sector and the government. Everyone knows someone in the office who lingered in a prominent job as their faculties declined—the one who became the subject of lunchtime gossip and averted eyes. But it's no longer just that person in the corner office, overly ego-invested in his job. There won't be enough generous retirement packages for the huge demographic swath of those people on the horizon. Anticipate a spate of disgruntled workers, management struggles, lawsuits, as well as the sporadic incident of workplace violence when things really go haywire.

Both the public and private sectors will require procedures providing oversight when somebody can no longer do their job. Currently that function is filled by mandatory retirement policies. In places like Congress where there is no mandatory retirement age, Strom Thurmond and his associates can stay on far longer than they should. But in many large corporations, mandatory retirement is simply a necessary but blunt instrument designed to permit the company to anticipate future personnel costs. It doesn't always identify the workers incapable of functioning effectively and often works perversely the other way. Many people now reaching mandatory retirement age between fifty-five and sixty-five are healthier than those of past generations, still able to do their jobs, and unable to transfer their skills to other occupations once they are retired.

Enter the medical profession—physicians, psychologists, social workers, and other professionals specializing in neurologic and occupational evaluation. They will play an important role in the future, not only as caregivers but also as consultants to business and government, expert witnesses in lawsuits, and as go-betweens to mediate disputes between workers who want to remain in their positions and employers wanting to let them go.

These medical professionals will have a host of new evaluation tools at their disposal—an emerging array of new imaging scanners of the central nervous system, individual genetic information, and evolving research on the diverse and often-unpredictable patterns of aging. Their collective judgment will play an integral role in American society as the baby boomers leave the workforce.

William Shakespeare described the tragedy of the impaired elderly as they exit the public stage in one of the supreme works in the English language, *King Lear*. The old and once-powerful king, in "the infirmity of his age," divided his kingdom unwisely—an incomprehensible act no one was willing to challenge. This fateful decision ultimately led to war in his kingdom, his death, and that of his children.

A preferable real-life model, sans tragedy, is that of famous American essayist Ralph Waldo Emerson, who developed severe dementia in his late sixties and could no longer write or lecture. In neurologist Oliver Sacks's bestseller *Musicophilia*, he described how Emerson retained his sense of irony and humor. When asked how he felt, even in his state of advanced dementia, Emerson would smile and answer, "Quite well; I have lost my mental faculties but am perfectly well." For those who can no longer pursue their lives' work, assuring retirement at the right time and making sure they are happy should be the goal of an enlightened society.

VI

PAST EPIDEMICS
AND FUTURE THREATS

51

WHEN THE CLIMATE CHANGES, SO DOES HEALTH

Almost daily and in every part of the world, new health
hazards arise from modern technology. Some of these hazards
make an immutable public impact. . . . Others attract less
attention because they lack the drama and are not obvious in
their effects. . . . Such is the case for the dangers posed
by certain pollutants of air, water and food, which remain almost
unnoticed despite their potential importance for public health. . . .
Hardly anything is known of the delayed effects of pollutants
on human life, even though they probably constitute
the most important threats to health in the long run.

—RENÉ JULES DUBOS

WHEN RENÉ JULES DUBOS, a professor of tropical medicine at
Harvard and a Pulitzer Prize winner, wrote those words in 1965,
the world had never heard of the terms *global warming* and *climate change*.
Today, with climate change a prominent political, social, and scientific

issue, it behooves us to pay heed to the warning Dubos issued nearly fifty years ago. Future policy debates should incorporate the potential effects and future likelihood of the international health consequences of global climate change.

When it comes to the health of individuals and societies, the relationship between man and nature has always been a tenuous one. Massive plagues and epidemics have devastated entire societies and have continually changed the course of history. Disease played a prominent role in the Peloponnesian War, striking down nearly a third of the population of Periclean Athens (including Pericles himself) during its war with Sparta in 429 BC. In the Middle Ages, the black death (bubonic plague) killed off one-third of the population of Europe.

The sixteenth-century Spanish conquest of Mexico by Hernán Cortés, which changed the face of Mesoamerica, may not have been possible had it not been for a smallpox epidemic that killed thousands of Aztec warriors during the battle in 1520 for the Aztec capital, Tenochtitlan. In the last century, an influenza epidemic at the end of World War I took as many as thirty million or more lives throughout the world in one year, far more than all the combat casualties of the actual war itself. Since the 1970s, AIDS has been an international scourge, killing millions, and even today millions of people die every year of AIDS and other communicable diseases on the African and Asian subcontinents.

Nor are infectious diseases the only natural disasters to have killed millions and radically altered societal patterns. The European Little Ice Age of the thirteenth and fourteenth centuries was devastating to the indigenous inhabitants of northern Europe and caused mass migrations across the continent. China has historically been afflicted with terrible river flooding, which has killed millions over the centuries. Drought, a natural calamity in much of central Africa and Australia, has periodically decimated and displaced entire populations of those continents.

Today the world faces another potential threat—the adverse health consequences of climate change and global warming. At the outset it should be noted that the climate variability that may result in a warmer world in the next century is certainly the way global temperatures are trending, but there is no uniform agreement about how quickly or how much the Earth will warm (a difference of even one degree Celsius would change factors such as insect-vector spread). Further, the debate extends to how much of that warming is the direct result of rising concentrations of atmospheric greenhouse gases due to the burning of fossil fuels and other human activities (scientific estimates range from a slight contribution to over 100 percent, the latter suggesting the Earth would otherwise be cooling). Finally, there is debate as to what measures should be taken—primarily an economic and political, rather than a scientific issue.

What is clear is that the Earth's surface temperatures have been warming steadily for the past eight decades (coincident with rising carbon dioxide concentrations), although there is a suggestion that the warming trend, while continuing to rise, may have slowed slightly in the last decade (this is according to the Goddard Institute for Space Studies and Climate Research Unit). If the warming trend of the current generation does continue unabated in the next century, it presents a number of serious potential health consequences. Anticipating these health risks will allow us to take action to prevent the catastrophic social, demographic, and economic upheaval that could result worldwide.

Because climate is such a complex phenomenon, it is difficult to predict precisely how climatic changes could affect human health. Moreover, all the changes may not be adverse; some may even be beneficial—for example, the health effects of milder winters in some areas might mitigate some of the effects of hotter summers in others. Assuming overall warmer temperatures worldwide, there will be associated changes in precipitation, humidity, and wind patterns. We can anticipate the concomitant health effects as likely to fall into three categories: increases in extreme weather events, infectious diseases primarily due to water and insect transmission, and changes in the ecosystem that affect food supply. Not surprisingly the most profound effects of all these would probably be seen in the world's poorer populations.

Extreme Weather Events

Climate change is often misunderstood to mean simply warming of the environment. Weather variability—that is, shifts in day-to-day conditions— is also a possible consequence of climate change. Even a small increase in mean temperatures in the coming decades, if accompanied by an increase in the variability of weather patterns, could result in a rise in the frequency of extremely hot days to dangerous levels. (Consider what would happen in Chicago if the average summer high temperature, currently 85 degrees, increased almost imperceptibly to 87, but the number of days at least five degrees higher than average doubled from the current eighteen. Instead of eighteen days with temperatures above 90 degrees, there would now be thirty-six days with temperatures above 92. Dangerous heat waves would become a routine occurrence.) An increased number of heat waves could pose a serious threat to many countries, especially those where populations are aging and moving to urban areas.

Currently, roughly half the world's population is located in cities, but by 2030 this figure is expected to increase to 60 percent. Because of roads, buildings, and industry, large cities tend to be "heat islands" that can reach temperatures ten to twelve degrees higher than the surrounding country-side (in Chicago, Lake Michigan modifies this effect). The Chicago heat wave of 1995 killed over seven hundred people, and a 2003 heat wave in southern France may have killed as many as fifteen thousand people, with mortality occurring primarily in the elderly, the infirm, and those socially isolated. It is not clear that either of these heat events was the result of global warming; both could have been isolated weather events. Nevertheless they illustrate the devastating potential for heat-related mortality in future extreme weather events.

Besides heat-related mortality, climate change poses the threat of deaths from the increased frequency and severity of storms, especially hurricanes in the Atlantic, typhoons in the Pacific, and cyclones in the Indian Ocean, as well as smaller-scale storms such as tornadoes in the American Midwest. Deaths from flooding, wind damage, and waterborne disease are all potential consequences. Hurricane Katrina in 2006, a storm that was an isolated weather event and probably not a consequence of global warming, did immense damage as a result of its strike over a populated land mass and the resultant storm surge. Global predictive models are still not sophisticated enough to forecast the likelihood of similar future storms, but the threat, while uncertain, remains real.

Infectious Diseases

Even a mild increase in temperatures, especially in the tropics, will increase the incidence and seasonal transmission of various infectious diseases by extending the geographic range of vector hosts such as insects, ticks, and water snails. These disease carriers are the intermediate hosts for a number of serious conditions, including malaria, Lyme disease, sleeping sickness, yellow fever, viral encephalitis, and West African river blindness.

Malaria is a case in point. Mathematical models have demonstrated that changes in rainfall patterns and temperature could allow the mosquitoes that transmit the disease to flourish and drastically increase the number of people exposed in endemic areas of Africa. Malaria was common in Europe in the nineteenth century and was still seen in southern Europe as recently as the 1950s. It is conceivable that, with climate change, the European continent could see a recurrence, especially if the mosquito vector demonstrates resistance to the insecticides currently used for control.

After a period of decline in the middle of the last century, African sleeping sickness, trypanosomiasis, now kills forty thousand people in central Africa annually. A warming of less than five degrees (Fahrenheit) would permit the tsetse fly, the insect vector, to disperse southward. Were the fly able to extend its geographical boundary as far south as South Africa, the disease could threaten the large livestock reserves and population centers of that country. Another potential infectious disease threat is cholera, which can be rapidly fatal in its most severe forms and is currently found in Asia,

Africa, South America, Central America, and Mexico. There were several serious cholera outbreaks in the United States in the nineteenth century. The causative organism may be harbored in oceanic coastal waters, and some believe that if sea surface temperatures were to increase, the bacterium would proliferate, causing major cholera epidemics worldwide.

Food Supply

Changes in precipitation patterns and temperature could have a profound effect on regional food yields and water supplies (imagine the implications if climate change caused a dislocation of the abundant midwestern American corn and soybean production several hundred miles north to southern Canada). Any shifts in food production would be unpredictable, but in some areas, drought and heat would likely result in widespread malnutrition and contaminated water supplies. Diseases like tuberculosis and typhoid could become endemic. Refugees from affected areas would flood toward areas with more food, cleaner and more accessible water, and better opportunities for employment. It is not hard to imagine population migration scenarios resulting in the increased spread of disease and even the possibility of armed conflicts.

Nor would the problem be confined to land-based agriculture. Countries such as Japan that depend primarily on fish as their dietary staple might be affected by changes in fluctuations in ocean temperatures. Changes in ocean currents and the warmth of the water could change the locations where fish reside. Moreover, there is some evidence that these factors would also increase the uptake of pollutants like mercury in the fish that constitute a vital part of the food chain.

There are a host of uncertainties about whether the worst effects of climate change and global warming will actually occur. Despite the most complicated mathematical models currently available, the future remains a mystery. But even if a mild degree of global warming should take place over the next generation, the possibility of the aforementioned effects on human health suggests certain strategies to mitigate or avoid worst-case scenarios.

Every scientific discipline has a role. Epidemiologists should be concentrating on case surveillance for serious infectious diseases while the public health community strengthens public health defenses and adopts strategies such as mosquito control and netting campaigns. Meanwhile, medical scientists must develop new vaccines and prevention campaigns for serious infectious diseases. Plant biologists must work on developing new crops resistant to drought and disease while meteorologists work on more precise models to predict severe weather events such as hurricanes and heat waves. Local and national governments should be involved in issues such as water conservation and purification, as well as measures to protect their citizens in the event of health emergencies.

Ironically, René Dubos was prescient in articulating the threat to human health from the delayed effects of pollutants long before the current concern about climate change. So perhaps it is not surprising that Dubos, who almost certainly knew nothing of the issue of global warming, is credited by many as the original author of one of the famous maxims that still applies to the debate—"Think globally, act locally."

52

ZIKA: THE LATEST EXOTIC TRAVELER TO STIR UP TROUBLE

Variability is the law of life, and as no two faces are the same,
so no two bodies are alike, and no two individuals react alike
and behave alike under abnormal conditions
which we know as disease.

—Sir William Osler, MD

I N ANCIENT TIMES, bacteria and viruses could not travel between different countries and regions faster than humans could migrate on foot. Distant populations were relatively safe from foreign diseases. The transmissibility of disease expanded tremendously when travel by horse, and then ship, became common.

With the twentieth-century development of intercontinental jet travel, global trade, tourism, and human migration, the "new normal" is epidemics and exotic diseases that can travel faster, farther, and in larger numbers than ever before in history. Witness the mosquito-borne Zika virus, which was barely on the World Health Organization's radar and then suddenly ravaged South America, with thousands infected.

Zika infection is usually not life threatening; however, it may occasionally be associated with the severe neurological condition Guillain-Barre syndrome. And health officials now believe Zika has a connection to microcephaly, a birth defect that can lead to severe brain damage. An alarming number of women who contracted Zika while pregnant have delivered babies with microcephaly. There is currently no vaccine or cure for Zika infection.

Readiness is everything. Recall that a Dallas hospital, as a result of bureaucracy and inadequate preparation, misdiagnosed the first case of Ebola virus in the United States in a patient traveling from Liberia. The infected patient was released from the hospital but returned three days later, and by then it was too late. He subsequently died. Two nurses who had contact with him contracted the virus, and nearly 150 people had to be monitored for six weeks. Fortunately, Ebola is not easily transmissible; otherwise the situation could easily have been disastrous.

The history of the Western Hemisphere is replete with examples of deadly contagions brought from distant parts of the world. While most transmission of exotic diseases today is from less developed countries to more developed ones, it was not always so. In the Middle Ages, smallpox was unknown to the Native American tribes. Ships with the first European settlers brought the disease, killing a large percentage of Native Americans in what is now the United States and Canada. Smallpox was also critical to the Spanish conquest of the Aztec and Inca empires of Mexico and South America.

In the eighteenth century, yellow fever, originating in either Africa or Central America, ravaged the major port cities of the eastern United States. In the nineteenth century, cholera, brought from Central Asia to England and ultimately by ship to America, caused epidemics in urban areas, including Chicago (federal troops sent via the Great Lakes to fight the Black Hawk War brought cholera to the city). The successful battles to control cholera and yellow fever are two of the underappreciated heroic stories in American history.

The influenza pandemic of 1918 was the country's worst infectious disease catastrophe. It is estimated that one-quarter of all Americans contracted the virus, and in only one year, an estimated 675,000 died, ten times as many as in World War I. The epidemic was fueled by the return of American soldiers who contracted the disease in Europe. Ships carrying returning doughboys and wounded veterans were a virtual incubation laboratory for the influenza virus.

Later in the twentieth century, the United States fortunately avoided an epidemic of avian influenza (bird flu), caused by a related influenza virus that originated in south China. Today the greatest fear of epidemiologists and infectious disease experts is the prospect of another lethally mutating influenza virus.

In our generation, the deadliest American epidemic has been AIDS, and the responsible virus, HIV, originated in central Africa. The HIV virus has been responsible for nearly as many American deaths as the 1918 influenza pandemic virus, albeit over a forty-year period. Since the beginning of the twenty-first century, the United States has also faced threats from the SARS virus, which originated in China, and the West Nile virus, first identified in East Africa. In all of these cases, the spread to America was abetted by global air travel moving infected victims or aircraft and ships moving mosquitoes or mosquito eggs.

We cannot roll back the clock on global travel and trade or their consequences. The Zika virus is merely the latest, but not the last, reminder of how advances in transportation leave us susceptible to once-unimaginable diseases. Luck is essential to avoiding these epidemics, but a famous scientific aphorism reminds us that chance favors the prepared mind. This will mean heightened levels of national and international preparation, including increased mosquito control, accelerated vaccine research, and advanced computer-assisted disease mapping and contact tracing.

53

EBOLA: HUMILITY IN THE FACE OF NATURE IS ESSENTIAL

The perpetual enemies of the human race,
apart from man's own nature, are ignorance and disease.

—ALAN GREGG, MD

I N THE RESPONSE TO EBOLA, the medical community quickly addressed its initial errors, which included the failure to promptly diagnose the first domestic case in Dallas and the inadequate protocol for caregivers. Lapses of this sort aren't likely to happen again. But what remains is an attitude from government officials that is sometimes condescending, bordering on arrogant. What message did the public receive when officials said they had no doubt they would stop Ebola in its tracks? Or when they quickly blamed a Dallas nurse for getting infected by breaching protocol, when the protocol was unclear?

During both the AIDS epidemic in the 1980s and the 1976 swine flu episode that really never materialized as an epidemic, the rhetoric of government officials damaged their credibility. To avoid a repeat of those missteps, officials should heed the following lessons from those medical crises:

1. *Avoid patronizing the public.* The unequivocal message delivered to the American public regarding Ebola was "don't panic." This is the right message, but the delivery of that message has frequently been the equivalent of a patronizing pat on the head. Rather than an admonishment, "don't panic" should be an exhortation to the public. During the Great Depression, when President Franklin D. Roosevelt told Americans not to panic over the parlous economic environment, he used the famous phrase "The only thing we have to fear is fear itself." He was exhorting citizens to engage in a communal effort, unencumbered by panic. That should be how officials reassure the public about Ebola.

2. *Tell us what you know—and what you don't know.* We have limited experience with Ebola. There is a reasonably good understanding of how Ebola is transmitted; the risk of transmission is virtually negligible from an asymptomatic patient who is not shedding a large amount of virus. Some officials and journalists say Ebola is "hard to get." By itself this means little. Hard, compared with what? It is quite hard to become infected with Ebola compared with exposure to measles or certain strains of influenza. But Ebola is obviously not that hard to get if you are caring for a patient; it is certainly easier than acquiring HIV during caregiving.

3. *Understand and deal with the limitations of information.* Computerized models are being used to analyze past Ebola outbreaks and are critically important to understanding how Ebola will spread in the future. But every model is based on finite information and is an imperfect predictor. Models also fail to account for human frailty—for example, an exposed health care worker who decides to fly—or unpredictable events like natural disasters or political instability in a stricken country. In contrast our ability to gather information is exponentially better than it was for the early years of the AIDS epidemic. The private information companies like Google and Apple should be enlisted to employ their information retrieval expertise

in West Africa and gather data on viral migration patterns and details on affected populations.

4. *Exude humility, not arrogance.* In the future those infected with Ebola are likely to be identified and isolated quickly. So long as the reservoir of infected people is small, and their contact is casual and limited, widespread transmission is unlikely. However, if those infected circulate with more people and have longer and more intimate contact, the chance of viral spread increases.

Hospitals were the initial focal point of transmission in the United States, and spread was contained. Whether there will be a future danger in large gathering places (subways, stadiums, airports) remains an unknown. Ultimately the key to preventing a pandemic will be eradicating Ebola in West Africa. The late Nobel Prize winner Joshua Lederberg, one of the world's leading experts in molecular biology, once observed that a microbe that felled a child in a distant continent yesterday can reach ours today and seed a global pandemic tomorrow. He warned, "The human race evidently has withstood the pathogenic challenges encountered so far, albeit with episodes of incalculable tragedy. But the rules of encounter and engagement have been changing; the same record of survival may not necessarily hold for the future."

Humility, in the face of nature, is essential.

54

MEASLES: A NEVER-ENDING THREAT

It can be said that each civilization has a pattern
of disease peculiar to it. The pattern of disease is an expression of
the response of man to his total environment (physical, biological,
social); this response is, therefore, determined by anything
that affects man himself or his environment.

—René Jules Dubos

THE DESERTED GRAVEYARD called Vunivesi sits silently by a small brook obscured by a mangrove canopy on the South Sea island of Fiji. The mass gravesite, abandoned decades ago, is unknown even to most Fijians. No one knows how many are buried there, but many of the dead likely spent their final moments lying in the nearby water for relief from fever and suffering.

Across the Pacific Ocean, five thousand miles away, are the trendy West Los Angeles enclaves of Santa Monica, Brentwood, and Beverly Hills, among the world's wealthiest communities. What could these affluent neighborhoods possibly have in common with the quiet graveyard of Vunivesi?

Measles.

In 1875 one of deadliest outbreaks of measles in modern history devastated Fiji, killing one-third of the island's one hundred thousand inhabitants. Ironically, measles was Fiji's first gift from Great Britain upon becoming a member of the British Empire. To celebrate Fiji's entrance into the Commonwealth, a British ship escorted Fijian leaders for a state visit to Sydney, Australia, then the closest British government seat. The entourage stayed at Sydney's finest hotel, amazed by the conveniences of the modern world. Unfortunately, they were also infected by a measles epidemic coursing through eastern Australia. They carried the disease back to Fiji, and within weeks measles swept over the island, killing thousands.

One medical historian wrote, "Death drums sounded incessantly in seemingly deserted villages. So many died so quickly that timely burial became impossible. Graves were only half dug because no one had the strength to dig." Lacking the strength to find food, thousands more died of starvation. After the outbreak, one British missionary described the eerie stillness of the deserted villages.

One hundred and forty-three years is not that long ago. Many baby boomers' great-grandparents, and some grandparents, could have been born around 1875. Among America's greatest achievements in that time has been the near eradication of vaccine-preventable diseases. The numbers for measles are impressive; in the pre-vaccine year of 1958, there were 763,094 cases and 552 deaths. In 2004 there were thirty-seven cases—a historical low—and not a single measles death was reported. But measles is making a comeback, and one of the "hot zones" is Southern California. Researching the story, the *Hollywood Reporter* found

the local children statistically at the greatest risk for infection aren't, as one might imagine, the least privileged—far from it. An examination by *The Hollywood Reporter* of immunization records submitted to the state by educational facilities suggests that wealthy Westside kids—particularly those attending exclusive, entertainment-industry-favored child care centers, preschools and kindergartens—are far more likely to get sick (and potentially infect their siblings and playmates) than other kids in LA.

The reason is at once painfully simple and utterly complex: More parents in this demographic are choosing not to vaccinate their children against the advice of medical experts. They express their noncompliance by submitting a form known as a personal belief exemption instead of paperwork documenting a completed shot schedule. . . . [In some schools] numbers are in line with immunization rates in developing countries like Chad and South Sudan.

The current anti-vaccine movement had its roots in a 1998 study by a British doctor, Andrew Wakefield. His now-discredited study was published in the world's most prestigious medical journal, the *Lancet*. The *Lancet* retracted the paper after discovering Wakefield's methods were sloppy and unethical, his conclusions unwarranted, and that he had failed to disclose significant financial interests. The UK General Medical Council declared he acted dishonestly and irresponsibly. Despite this, celebrities including Jenny McCarthy, Kristin Cavallari, and Robert Kennedy Jr. have spearheaded the anti-vaccine movement.

This marks a dramatic reversal from a time when Hollywood celebrities enthusiastically endorsed the fight against polio. In 1956, at the height of his popularity, Elvis Presley posed for his polio vaccination. Parents, witnessing the tragedy of death and paralysis, lined up to have their children inoculated with the still incompletely tested polio vaccine. The medical community must exert greater leadership. The former surgeon general Vivek Murthy, having been out of residency for less than a decade, may have lacked historical perspective when he said tentatively: "The most important message I have is to please, please, please get your child vaccinated. . . . I recognize that some of the concerns parents have about vaccinations come from a place of wanting to do the best to protect their children. . . . I believe that on this topic, the science is very clear."

No mention of the lax immunization requirements in states like California. Murthy's comments, like those of Republican presidential hopefuls Rand Paul and Chris Christie, may be tempered by political concerns. But Murthy should have drawn from the example of one of his predecessors, C. Everett Koop. Koop, surgeon general during the early years of the AIDS epidemic, infuriated many conservative supporters with candid, medically accurate statements about HIV. He was forceful and undeterred by politics. "Everything I ever said caused controversy," he said. "That's the nature of the job. . . . It's a controversial job and you have to have a very thick skin, and you cannot let yourself be pushed by political pressures about what is politically correct and what is not."

Right now that type of candor is needed. Those unfortunate Fijians at Vunivesi were victims of something they were unaware of and could not control. If future Americans fall victim to a severe strain of measles or another vaccine-preventable disease, then, in the words of William Shakespeare, we will have failed to "take arms against a sea of troubles and by opposing end them."

55

ANTI-VAXXERS

Disease is a fate of the poor, but also a punishment of the rich.
—IVO ANDRIC, NOBEL LAUREATE IN LITERATURE

ANTI-VAXXERS IS THE TWENTY-FIRST-CENTURY TERM that refers to those who oppose vaccination in preventing infectious diseases. Regrettably it's only a matter of time before this new term enters the *Oxford English Dictionary*. During the 2016 presidential campaign, the issue went mainstream when two major candidates, Jill Stein and Donald Trump, neither an overt anti-vaxxer, both went on record as being at least somewhat suspicious of the vaccine process.

No longer a small band of cranks, anti-vaxxers are an organized group who proselytize in communities across the country—with effect. They certainly bear some responsibility for the recent measles outbreak in Minnesota, where there were at least sixty-nine cases, primarily children, with more than ten hospitalized. The majority of Minnesota cases have occurred in the Somali community, which has been actively targeted by the anti-vaxxers.

David Johnson, program manager with the Hennepin County Health Department, told NBC News,

> What we have now is a community that was really influenced by these anti-vaccine groups. And they've performed a natural experiment: to forgo the measles vaccine based on this propaganda. . . . There has been ongoing contact between outside groups who have come in and wanted to do organizing within the community that's affected here . . . and I think that's really unfortunate because some of the anti-vaccine propaganda is largely to blame for what's going on in our community. . . . They've preyed on parents' concerns about the health of their children and they've provided them false hope that avoiding the measles vaccine will somehow prevent autism, when in fact not vaccinating only serves to increase the risk of a child getting a disease and then spreading it to others.

The anti-vaxxers do not confine their activities to immigrant communities. After a Disneyland outbreak of measles in 2015 that spread to seven states, Canada, and Mexico, a study revealed that some of the highest levels of vaccine skepticism and lowest levels of vaccination occurred in communities of largely graduate-level educated residents in affluent California counties.

With decades of overwhelming scientific evidence supporting vaccination and countless lives saved, how did the anti-vaxxers gain such traction? Ironically it was partly the success of vaccine programs in eradicating childhood diseases that were once fatal or that caused severe brain damage. The thinking goes, Why take a chance and vaccinate my child for a disease he or she won't get or at worst will cause nothing more than a rash?

History has also played a role. The infamous Tuskegee Study, which played out from 1932 to 1972, saw public health officials withhold treatment from poor rural African American farmers in Alabama as part of an observational study of syphilis. This had a long-lasting effect in undermining confidence in the medical community, especially among minorities.

Likewise, the government and physicians lost credibility during the swine flu debacle of 1976, when officials drastically overestimated the chances of a swine flu pandemic and failed to anticipate a small but significant number of neurologic side effects of vaccination during a national immunization program.

The most egregious vaccination problem was the Cutter incident when polio gripped the United States in the early 1950s. Jonas Salk and his team developed a vaccine from inactivated poliovirus, and after testing they found it to be effective in hundreds of thousands of children nationwide. However, during the subsequent national immunization campaign in 1955, two hundred thousand children received a batch of defective vaccine manufactured at Cutter Laboratories in which live virus was still present. Thousands of polio cases were reported, two hundred children were left paralyzed, and ten died.

Some sources blamed the incident on Cutter, while others blamed the federal government for inadequate oversight. Julius Youngner, the last surviving member of the Salk team and one of the last people with direct experience with the Cutter incident, died recently, blaming Dr. Salk to the end for not preventing the tragedy (the two men had a falling out, which undoubtedly colored Youngner's account).

Whatever the cause, the episode led to greater federal regulation of vaccines. Ironically, there was no public hesitation to receive the polio vaccine when it was reintroduced; back then we lived in a far less skeptical world.

Today virtually every study has failed to find any link between vaccines and autism. Just as important is the documented effectiveness of vaccines. When the grandparents of today's parents were children, death from childhood diseases was a grim presence in every American community. According to the Centers for Disease Control and Prevention (CDC), in 1900 there were 21,064 smallpox cases and 894 deaths. There were 469,924 measles cases and 7,575 deaths in 1920, as well as 147,991 diphtheria cases and 13,170 deaths. In 1922 there were 107,473 pertussis cases and 5,099 deaths. Now vaccination has virtually eliminated these deaths.

Nevertheless, the anti-vaxxers are not going away. The most that can be done to counter them is better communication of reliable information by journalists and the health care community, along with a tightening of state laws making personal exemptions, a loophole anti-vaxxers commonly exploit, harder to obtain. After the Disneyland measles epidemic, the California State Legislature introduced more rigorous legislation regarding personal exemptions.

In our modern society, anti-vaxxers have taught us a tragic lesson: namely that better information, combined with more experience and more knowledge, does not always translate into greater wisdom.

56

WHEN THE AVIAN FLU COMES

In the whole the face of things, as I say, was much altered;
sorrow and sadness sat upon every face; and though some parts
were not yet overwhelmed, yet all looked deeply concerned;
and as we saw it apparently coming on, so everyone looked
on himself and his family as in the utmost danger.

—DANIEL DEFOE, *A JOURNAL OF THE PLAGUE YEAR*

CONSIDER THIS SCENARIO: A duck migrating through China stops to inspect a chicken that has died of avian flu, and the duck contracts the flu virus. The duck then carries the virus to a farm in Hong Kong and infects pigs, which already harbor a human flu virus, contracted from the farm's owner. The pigs become the ideal breeding ground for a virulent hybrid virus created by the shuffling of genetic material between human and bird viruses. The lethal hybrid virus is passed to the farmer and quickly appears in Hong Kong.

A month later the boss greets you and coworkers entering the company's conference room for a morning meeting. He distributes handouts

as he tells stories about his recent Far East vacation. He has a brief cough-
ing spell.

The convergence of the events in the Far East and that morning meeting
means the boss's innocent cough might convert that conference room into
a deadly source of contagion for employees, their families, and their friends.

The irony of human epidemics is that they usually begin in a subtle,
innocuous fashion—something to ponder when you read about the prospects of a future avian flu epidemic. During flu season, most of the emphasis
is on what the government will or won't do to control such an epidemic.
But the private sector must expand its role in controlling and managing this
threat too. The entire workforce has to develop a heightened consciousness.

The United Nation's World Health Organization has predicted that
between 2 million and 7.4 million people could die from a global influenza
pandemic if one occurred today. The economic costs could potentially
run into the hundreds of billions of dollars. Quarantine would be a real
possibility, causing serious social disruption. President George W. Bush
once even proposed using the US military to contain a flu outbreak. The
government is constantly working on vaccine testing and developing and
acquiring large stocks of antiviral drugs.

But Hurricane Katrina taught us the folly of putting all our eggs in
the government's basket—government can only do so much. If a lethal flu
strain did happen to strike, even a perfect response by federal, state, and
local government would not avert disaster. Reliance on the public sector
alone would be insufficient. Early involvement of the private sector will be
imperative for economic preservation and, more important, to save lives.

Even before flu season arrives, the first step by companies should be
the pedestrian, but absolutely essential, provision of providing tissues (in
some settings, face masks) and hand sanitizers to employees. Hand hygiene
should be a priority. It's important to encourage employees to get a flu
vaccine; the strains the flu vaccine is most effective against every year are
more likely than the avian flu to cause human disease, so it is a reasonable
approach.

Second, when a flu outbreak occurs, contagion is such a threat that employees should be encouraged not to come to work if they develop flu-like symptoms. This means companies may have to allow more sick days. Whenever possible work should be done at home and conferencing should be online; the flu virus is one virus the Internet won't transmit. Businesses where an epidemic increases foot traffic, such as pharmacies, emergency medical services, and health care facilities, should have replacement workers on call.

Conversely, in the event of a severe outbreak, businesses such as entertainment sites and nonessential retail stores should anticipate temporary shutdowns. Finally, private businesses have a critical role in working with public health officials to provide information and reassurance to a worried public in the event of a possible epidemic. And some legal indemnification may be necessary. Businesses, by suppressing their inherent aversion to government requests, could perform a service by providing important surveillance information on employees' health status to government authorities.

In the worst-case situation, an avian flu outbreak could create social dislocation and suffering unknown in the United States since the 1918 influenza pandemic. The personal toll on every citizen would be incalculable. To spare us a similar fate, the private sector must be part of any comprehensive national plan on how to deal with avian flu and other contagious strains.

57

THE CHICAGO EXPERIENCE
WITH A NINETEENTH-CENTURY
EPIDEMIC THAT KILLS
AGAIN TODAY

The human mind always tries to expunge the intolerable from memory, just as it tries to conceal it while current.

—H. L. MENCKEN

A CHOLERA EPIDEMIC that began in 2010 has devastated Haiti, killing nearly ten thousand people and hospitalizing tens of thousands. The epidemic is still not completely under control in the country, with several hundred new infections each month. Meanwhile, in 2017 a cholera epidemic emerged in war-torn Yemen; there have been over one hundred thousand cases and over one thousand deaths.

Cholera, caused by a waterborne bacterium, thrives in areas of unsanitary conditions, overcrowding, and shortages of clean water. It results in diarrhea and rapidly fatal dehydration unless treated promptly with fluids and antibiotics. The Haitian epidemic resulted from the aftermath of tropical storms and a devastating earthquake. But officials have acknowledged it was also the result of inadvertent contamination by UN peacekeepers. It is a reminder that cholera, a pandemic disease in the nineteenth century, can still ravage the twenty-first-century Third World.

Because improved sanitation and modern medicine have drastically reduced the threat of cholera in the industrialized world, few remember its impact on the United States two centuries ago. Major European and American cities, including Chicago, were plagued by successive cholera epidemics, causing tens of thousands of deaths. Because Chicago developed along Lake Michigan, its early history was profoundly influenced by those outbreaks, and vestiges of that influence remain today.

Until 1816 cholera was a disease limited to South Asia. The first cholera epidemic remained contained in eastern Asia until 1823. However, in 1826 a second Asian pandemic began, and cholera was carried by Russian troops into Poland in 1831. Within a year, the disease was endemic in Europe and the British Isles, devastating London and Paris. It spread as a by-product of the early Industrial Revolution. Steam-powered rapid transportation, urban population migration, crowded slums, inadequate water supplies, ineffective elimination of sewage, and unprepared city governments all played a part.

With trepidation Americans read in their newspapers of the European epidemic in the early 1830s. Inevitably, immigrants on crowded ships from Britain brought cholera to Montreal in 1831. Cholera crossed the St. Lawrence River and Great Lakes, cutting a swath through Buffalo, New York; Detroit, Michigan; and the Eastern Seaboard cities.

Cholera reached Chicago as a consequence of the 1832 Black Hawk War. Driven from Illinois, Chief Black Hawk, tribal leader of the Sauk and Fox, led a party from Iowa back across the Mississippi. The Illinois governor dispatched the Illinois militia and requested several thousand federal troops, who arrived on ships from Buffalo, commanded by Gen. Winfield Scott (future war hero of the Mexican-American War). This move was probably an overreaction since Black Hawk's "hostile war party" consisted of only one thousand, including six hundred women and children, who were bearing seeds for planting crops.

The Illinois militia quickly dispatched Black Hawk, ending forever the Native American threat to Cook County and the Chicago region. However, General Scott's troops, who proved unnecessary, brought cholera from Buffalo to Fort Dearborn, and hundreds died just before Chicago was incorporated in 1833.

The continuing threat of cholera was impetus for the creation of the Chicago Board of Health in 1835. Despite this, subsequent cholera epidemics broke out in 1845 (traveling up the Mississippi and brought by workers on the Illinois and Michigan Canal) and at least four other times before 1873, killing thousands of Chicagoans.

Those cholera epidemics were also responsible for Chicago's first hospitals, several small, temporary structures built in the 1840s and 1850s designed to isolate cholera and smallpox victims. Inadequate for Chicago's burgeoning population, they were replaced by Mercy Hospital, the oldest continuously running hospital in Chicago.

Today orphanages, homes for parentless children, are a little-remembered historical footnote. But they were once prominent institutions housing thousands in nineteenth-century Chicago. The first Chicago orphanages, the Chicago Orphan Asylum and the Catholic Orphan Asylum, began as a result of an 1849 cholera epidemic that left many children without parents. Social concerns caused orphanages to disappear eventually, but the eradication of cholera was one reason they were no longer necessary.

An 1851 cholera epidemic prompted the creation of Chicago's first public water board. The board commissioned an engineer with previous experience working on the Erie Canal to design a city water-supply system. The city's first water pipes were laid with a goal of preventing cholera and other diseases, as well as fighting fires in the wooden structures of the central business district (structures that burned during the infamous Great Chicago Fire of 1871).

The early burial grounds in Chicago were near Lake Michigan at Fort Dearborn, along the river. In the 1840s a large city cemetery complex extended in what is now Lincoln Park, including land the city purchased from the estate of a wealthy cholera victim. After another cholera epidemic, the proximity of the city cemetery to the water supply became a public health concern. In the 1860s, large numbers of bodies were transported to cemeteries farther from the lake, which remain today, including Graceland, Rosehill, and Oak Woods.

Improvements in sewage and sanitation finally ended the scourge of cholera in Chicago in the early 1880s. Over the years there were reports of a terrible 1885 epidemic of cholera and typhoid fever that killed ninety thousand. It is almost certainly an urban myth since no contemporaneous accounts exist, which would be incredible considering the improbably high number of deaths (equivalent to 250 Great Chicago Fires). By then cholera had basically been eradicated in Chicago.

Today cholera's impact on early Chicago has been largely forgotten. Barring a cataclysmic natural disaster or major societal upheaval, Chicagoans will never again experience a cholera epidemic. But the story of cholera is as integral to the fabric of Chicago as the colorful accounts of crooked politicians, World's Fairs, and gangsters that regale us in our history books.

VII

SCIENTIFIC PHILOSOPHY

58

CAN SCIENCE
AND RELIGION COEXIST?

Godspeed, John Glenn.

—Scott Carpenter

N 1962 PROJECT Mercury astronaut Scott Carpenter, the backup pilot
for *Friendship 7*, delivered one of the most famous phrases in American
history to pilot John Glenn, the first American to orbit the Earth. Ironically, Glenn never heard it because his microphone was tuned to a different frequency. Carpenter's message followed that of mission control test
conductor Tom O'Malley, who also broadcast a personal prayer, "May the
Good Lord ride all the way."

The significance of this story, beyond its historical importance, was the
underappreciated role of religion in the early American space program. Lost
in the eulogies for John Glenn when he died in 2016 was how important
religious faith was to him and some of his colleagues in the high-tech atmosphere of the space race. For a time Glenn and Buzz Aldrin, the second

man to walk on the moon, were elders in the same Houston church. A devout Presbyterian and churchgoer, Glenn prayed routinely during his flights as a test pilot and astronaut.

He once told the Associated Press that he saw no contradiction between belief in God and evolution: "I don't see that I'm any less religious by the fact that I can appreciate that science just records that we change with evolution and time. . . . It doesn't mean it's less wondrous and it doesn't mean that there can't be some power greater than any of us that has been behind and is behind whatever is going on."

In today's fractious secular society, such an opinion is not especially popular, particularly among scientists. The oft-quoted astrophysicist Neil deGrasse Tyson asserts publicly there is little common ground between science and religion. But besides John Glenn, there have always been men of science who have taken a more nuanced view of science and religion.

Dr. Charles Townes won the 1964 Nobel Prize in Physics for his invention of the laser and also the 2005 Templeton Prize for "exceptional contribution to affirming life's spiritual dimension, whether through insight, discovery, or practical works." (Dual winners of the Nobel and Templeton include Mother Teresa and the Dalai Lama.)

Dr. Townes once spoke of his religious belief in the context of outer space:

Science is an exploration of what things are like and how they work. Why they are that way is more a religious question. And the two are complementary. I think they are both important. Why did the universe begin? Why is the universe here? Why are we here? And why did the laws of science come out the way they are so we could be here. I think the apparent friction between science and religion is kind of artificial. I see no real friction between the two but some people want to make it that way. We need more integration between the two in the future. We need to be more open-minded and deeper in our thinking.

The world's greatest twentieth-century scientist, Albert Einstein, struggled his entire life with the fundamental relationship between religion and science. A secular Jew, Einstein abjured formal religion but disapproved of those who used his views to endorse atheism. He expressed a sentiment similar to Townes: "Science without religion is lame, religion without science is blind."

Richard Feynman, a giant of American physics and a celebrated iconoclast, delivered a famous speech in 1956 at the California Institute for Technology titled "The Relation of Science and Religion." Feynman, also a secular Jew, said, "Although science makes some impact on many religious ideas, it does not affect the moral content. Religion has many aspects; it answers all kinds of questions . . . about what things are, where they come from, what man is, what God is—the properties of God, and so on . . . the metaphysical aspect of religion."

Hardly a religious man, Feynman proceeded to raise the centuries-old question of the interplay of religion and science, which still resonates today:

> Religion also tells us another thing—how to behave. Leave out of this the idea of how to behave in certain ceremonies, and what rites to perform; I mean it tells us how to behave in life in general, in a moral way. It gives answers to moral questions; it gives a moral and ethical code. . . . Western civilization, it seems to me, stands by two great heritages. One is the scientific spirit of adventure—the adventure into the unknown, the attitude that all is uncertain; to summarize it—the humility of the intellect. The other great heritage is Christian ethics—the basis of action on love, the brotherhood of all men, the value of the individual—the humility of the spirit. These two heritages are logically, thoroughly consistent. But logic is not all; one needs one's heart to follow an idea. . . . How can we draw inspiration to support these two pillars of Western civilization so that they may stand together in full vigor, mutually unafraid? Is this not the central problem of our time?

As much as anyone, John Glenn understood the humility of the intellect. In 1998, at seventy-seven, he became the oldest man to go into space when he traveled on the space shuttle. When he returned, Glenn opined on Feynman's central problem, "To look out at this kind of creation and not believe in God is, to me, impossible. It just strengthens my faith."

Godspeed, John Glenn.

59

BACK TO THE FUTURE: NAVIGATING BY THE STARS

As technology goes up, creativity and imagination go down.

—JIM NICHOLSON

AS LONGTIME WRITER, reporter, and intelligence expert Jim Nicholson implies, technology should complement—not replace—old-school skills. In that vein, because of fears that the global positioning system (GPS) could be jammed or hacked, the US Navy has announced it will reinstitute classes on celestial navigation—that is, plotting course and direction by the stars. "We went away from celestial navigation because computers are great," Lt. Cmdr. Ryan Rogers, deputy chairman of the United States Naval Academy's department of seamanship and navigation, recently told the *Capital Gazette*. "The problem is there's no backup [for GPS]."

The navy will complement the more precise but potentially vulnerable GPS by teaching the navigation method mariners have employed since antiquity. The *New York Times* has reported that Russian submarines troll ominously close to critical undersea communication cables from the North Sea to waters near US shores, ready to disrupt high-tech communication, so this development represents a teachable moment about overreliance on technology.

If you've ever driven in a strange city or isolated area, you may be familiar with overdependence on technology. GPS is an invaluable tool that usually directs you reliably to your destination. But occasionally GPS will not tell you about detours and road construction or what the shortest route is. It may misidentify your destination and take you miles out of your way. So the value and reliability of GPS are enhanced by having a traditional paper map, the ability to read the map, and directions from local residents.

Societal progress results when each new generation acquires more information and greater knowledge and then constructs new tools to solve problems. But in the process, things are lost. So while knowledge increases in our modern society, fewer people know how to bake a cake from scratch, build a campfire, or read a map. Of course those skills no longer have much use, and if you really want to bake a cake, you can always google it. But the computer also creates a loss of knowledge, and the loss has been especially dramatic in skills acquired in childhood, such as cursive writing and spelling.

Another skill that is threatened is computational ability. Give a third grader a calculator to solve a list of math problems, and even with poor math skills, he or she will likely obtain the right answer for most problems. But the child will get some wrong, a few by a large margin. And without a math background, the child won't realize how bad their errors are: 12 x 10 is not 1,200. This matters and eventually becomes a more serious problem than just a generation that can't make change for a twenty-dollar purchase.

Medicine was confronted with a similar issue of technology versus experience in the 1980s. When CT scans were introduced, the technology facilitated making diagnoses that formerly required long hospital stays, dangerous procedures, or surgery. Today physicians routinely—sometimes too routinely—order CT scans as part of their immediate diagnostic plan.

This approach often results in an immediate diagnosis, albeit at a cost: new doctors fail to learn important skills, including how to take a history and examine a patient. If the CT scan does not, or cannot, provide the answer, the physicians are stymied. They are at a loss as to how to proceed.

The story of the CT scan provides a historical lesson about technology versus experience. When the first CT scans displayed images of the brain, some doctors predicted the technology would make neurologists obsolete. Others argued the opposite—the CT scan would never match an experienced neurologist doing a detailed history and physical. Ultimately, neither prediction proved true. CT scans revolutionized medicine and made all doctors better diagnosticians. The test did not make neurologists obsolete; good neurologists who knew how to interpret the test became even more valuable. What the introduction of the CT scan demonstrated was that experience plus technology is superior to either one alone. Today the challenge to the navy presented by GPS is similar to the one that medicine faced. Today's GPS is amazingly accurate, but guidance by the stars remains a necessary complementary technology. Capt. Timothy Tisch of the United States Merchant Marine Academy told the *Telegraph*, "Knowledge of celestial navigation in the GPS era provides a solid backup form of navigation in the event GPS becomes unreliable for whatever reason. It is also a good professional practice to use one navigational system to verify the accuracy of another."

This is a reminder that technology is invaluable for navigation, medical diagnosis, and teaching children math and verbal skills. However, and this is essential, without human experience GPS, CT scans, and tablet computers will never be sufficient to guarantee our future.

60

VOLKSWAGEN:
PRIMUM NON NOCERE

Primum non nocere (First, do no harm)

—A Hippocratic dictum

COMPUTER SOFTWARE NOW governs virtually every aspect of our lives, from cars to kitchen appliances; the human element has been removed from most machinery we use daily. But computer software can deceive us, and this was the disturbing message from the 2015 Volkswagen scandal, where the German carmaker fitted millions of cars with software that could outsmart emission-control testing. This demonstrates the need for a code of ethics, a Hippocratic oath, for our computer engineers and the software they create.

As part of an international campaign to market "clean" diesel vehicles, Volkswagen sold eleven million cars worldwide, nearly a half million in the United States, that were supposedly clean. They were not. The cars were equipped with "defeat devices," software that monitored variables including speed, engine features, and steering-wheel position, thus detecting when the car was undergoing emission testing.

During testing, the car immediately switched into a diminished power/performance mode that cut engine emissions sufficiently to pass the test. When the testing was completed, the car reverted to its normal driving mode, where pollutants far exceeded permissible levels. Once the deceptive software was developed and installed in cars, the scheme could be carried out without human involvement. By the same measure, it was virtually impossible for anyone unaware to uncover the deception (it was discovered serendipitously by professional engineers who were initially surprised by their findings).

The fallout from the scandal cost Volkswagen hundreds of millions of dollars, but the health costs to the public are incalculable. The nitrogen oxide pollutants released from the tainted vehicles aggravate the symptoms of people with asthma, bronchitis, emphysema, or heart disease. Some people will certainly die prematurely, even if the victims can never be directly linked to Volkswagen's subterfuge.

This scandal should begin a vigorous debate about the values that software developers incorporate in their software, not just in the automotive industry but in every industry. At present the public has little appreciation of the importance of software ethics. (What exactly does the familiar Google motto "Don't be evil" really mean?) Moreover, like law and medicine, the debate about software ethics appears to be a topic of discussion more in universities than in the real world.

This must change, and that's why what happened at Volkswagen is so important. Issues of safety, privacy, and confidentiality have to become essential professional concerns. The Volkswagen case should become a case study in every company that depends on software, as well as in the academic community.

Ethics for software engineers—what the public expects from the profession and what the profession expects from itself—will not replace the law but can complement it. Software engineers are less likely to cut corners if they know their behavior will earn the opprobrium of colleagues and engender public suspicion. Ignorance of the importance of software ethics is surely one more step in the descent into a more mistrustful society.

In a sense, the person who first brought the issue of software ethics to public attention was the brilliant scientist and science fiction author Isaac Asimov. In a 1942 magazine article, he developed the Three Laws of Robotics, a primitive code of behavior for robots, one applicable to today's software as well:

First Law: *A robot may not injure a human being, or through inaction, allow a human being to come to harm.*

Second Law: *A robot must obey the orders given by human beings, except where such orders would conflict with the First Law.*

Third Law: *A robot must protect its own existence, as long as such protection does not conflict with the First or Second Law.* (Asimov subsequently developed a Fourth Law that superseded the first three laws: A robot may not harm humanity, or, by inaction, allow humanity to come to harm. Volkswagen egregiously violated this law.)

When it came to malevolence, Asimov was hardly naive. He understood that the world was entering a new era of man and machine, one that would reveal uncharted territory of human behavior (so brazenly demonstrated by Volkswagen).

Asimov once said of his laws, "Whenever someone asks me if I think my Three Laws of Robotics will actually be used to govern the behavior of robots, once they become versatile and flexible enough to be able to choose among different courses of behavior, my answer is, 'Yes, the Three Laws are the only way in which rational human beings can deal with robots—or with anything else.' But when I say that, I always remember (sadly) that human beings are not always rational."

61

WHAT IS LIFE,
AND WHO IS CARL WOESE?

An honest man, armed with all the knowledge available to us now,
could only state that in some sense, the origin of life appears
at the moment to be almost a miracle, so many are the conditions
which would have had to have been satisfied to get it going.

—FRANCIS CRICK

LIFE IS HARD, as the philosophers love to remind us. Besides being
hard, life is also complex, as biology students soon learn when they
begin studying how living organisms are classified. So a little-known University of Illinois professor, Carl Woese, merits some recognition in that
respect. A giant in the science of biology who revolutionized the field,
Woese contributed a glorious chapter to the complexity of life.

From ancient times until recently in human history, classification of life
was simple: upon inspection a living thing was either an animal or a plant.
Then in the seventeenth century, Anton van Leeuwenhoek invented the

microscope and discovered bacteria invisible to the naked eye. This represented a fundamental problem for biology since these invisible organisms did not fall easily into either category of plant or animal.

Even as the legendary giants of biology, Charles Darwin and Carl Linnaeus, were refining biologic classification, no one had a clue how to classify bacteria for another two hundred years after the discovery of the microscope. In the nineteenth century, the centuries-old plant/animal paradigm forever changed when microscopic organisms were given their own place on the evolutionary life tree. At that point there were plants, animals, and then bacteria.

A new era in biology began in the twentieth century with the development of the electron microscope, an exponential development in technology. This new instrument permitted scientists to look at the cell nucleus and other subcellular structures. It became the tool by which biologists were able to refine their classifications of microorganisms.

Enter Carl Woese, who came of age professionally at the University of Illinois at Urbana-Champaign. While doing research early in his career, he took full advantage of another of the twentieth century's transformative events in biology—the discovery of DNA, genes, and genetic sequencing.

As befits great scientists who cross boundaries, Woese adapted these new discoveries to his own work, and the results were groundbreaking. Woese understood that living organisms no longer had to be classified by how they looked, as had been the case for centuries. Life, especially microorganisms, could now be classified by how their cells worked. By studying molecular structures, how cells manufacture proteins, and evaluating genetic sequences, Woese identified *Archaea*, a completely heretofore-undiscovered form of microbial life. Few scientists can lay claim to such a momentous discovery as a new life form.

Archaea are structurally and functionally different from common bacteria and represent a completely new branch on the evolutionary tree. They are believed to be the earliest forms of life (the word *Archaea* is Greek for "ancient"). *Archaea* were once thought to inhabit only extreme environments such as the Antarctic and suboceanic volcanoes. Now it is clear they are ubiquitous—in every climate and terrain, as well as in the human body.

It is a historical truism that great scientific discoveries often begin as heresies and rarely go unchallenged. Woese's description of a new life form was no exception. In the late 1970s, the scientific community did not immediately accept his published research on *Archaea*. It took two decades before he was vindicated and his discovery became a standard part of every biology textbook. Ironically, one of the signs of recognition he received from other biologists was his receipt of the 1992 Leeuwenhoek Medal, the top honor in microbiology. It is named after the man who, three centuries before, saw the first microbes under the microscope and whose work provided the foundation for Woese's work.

What is the significance of Carl Woese's discovery of *Archaea*? It is impossible to know all the implications; however, without question it will affect future generations. Most of *Archaea*'s functions are still unknown, but they play an important, albeit poorly understood, role in the regulation of gases in the Earth's atmosphere. In addition they afford a greater understanding of the origin of life on Earth and may provide a clue to whether life exists in outer space.

Someday some enterprising scientist, perhaps still to be born, will employ the knowledge Carl Woese gave us to investigate that question of extraterrestrial life.

Whatever happens, Woese's place is certified as one of the great transitional figures in evolutionary biology. Every scientist's work is the culmination of the work of the great scientists who came before him and a prologue to the chapters that will be written by those who follow him. So it was hardly an overstatement when one of Woese's colleagues told the journal *New Scientist* that Woese has done more for biology than any biologist in history—including Charles Darwin.

62

THE NFL MAY BECOME EXTINCT IF WE DO NOT PAY ATTENTION TO YOUTH FOOTBALL

———————

I am delighted to have you play football. I believe in rough, manly sports. But I do not believe in them if they degenerate into the sole end of any one's existence. I don't want you to sacrifice standing well in your studies to any over-athleticism; and I need not tell you that character counts for a great deal more than either intellect or body in winning success in life. Athletic proficiency is a mighty good servant, and like so many other good servants, a mighty bad master.

—THEODORE ROOSEVELT IN
THEODORE ROOSEVELT'S LETTERS TO HIS CHILDREN

THE NATIONAL FOOTBALL LEAGUE (NFL) may be as popular as ever, but when NFL immortals like Troy Aikman and Bo Jackson publicly announce they would never allow their children to play football, the game clearly faces an existential threat. Not since 1905, when President Theodore

Roosevelt rescued the game from its brutal, violent origins by demanding the outlaw of the dangerous strategy of players running downfield arms interlocked, the notorious "flying wedge," has the game's long-term future been in such peril.

Like other sports football must confront a litany of long-standing problems, including drug use by players, owners of dubious integrity, exorbitant salaries, franchises disloyal to home cities, uncertain television ratings, criminal behavior outside the lines, recruiting abuses, and labor difficulties.

But these problems, which come and go, are part and parcel of all professional sports. The existential threat to football, more than any other sport, is from head injuries and the concern of parents and younger players. If football is perceived to be unsafe, the pool of young players necessary to support a competitive NFL will eventually disappear.

After decades of denial, the NFL has finally admitted a direct connection between head trauma on the field and degenerative brain disease. The past decade has seen the premature retirement of current players, several suicides by retired players, class action lawsuits against the league, and settlement funds created to compensate injured players.

Meanwhile, youth football has witnessed an almost 10 percent drop in participation in the last eight years. Current research suggests that brain trauma in the young can stunt neurologic development and that earlier participation leads to a greater risk of long-term cognitive impairment. In addition even subconcussive blows can have a lasting negative impact. Understandably, parents across the country are increasingly uneasy about youth football.

Acknowledging these problem, USA Football, a group that sets standards for amateur football, has developed a plan to make youth football safer called Heads Up Football. Working with doctors and coaches, the group has made modifications in the game that include smaller playing fields, fewer players, and eliminating punts and kickoffs. Because the traditional head-down, one-hand stance places linemen in a vulnerable position, players are now instructed to position themselves in a heads-up crouch. Players are also taught to tackle and block with their heads up as well.

However, as Vince Lombardi observed, football is not a contact sport but a collision sport. In spite of these changes to the game, kids will still run into each other at full speed and hit one another as hard as they can. Head trauma will be reduced but not eliminated completely; concussions will still occur. But making the sport safer may assuage some parental fears and reduce player attrition.

As part of the process, USA Football is also promoting seven-on-seven flag football with no tackling, blocking, or full contact, so helmets are unnecessary. The focus is on promoting speed, coordination, and endurance that transfer to the next level. High school teams now regularly compete in seven-on-seven passing competitions that are essentially safe from the standpoint of head injuries.

There is no blocking and tackling in flag football, which makes it an especially attractive alternative for young players because those are the situations most conducive to head injuries. In truth, in youth football young players learn very little about blocking and tackling, which puts them at risk of serious injury, with no substantive value in terms of experience.

Most experts acknowledge that high school is the proper time to introduce players to full-contact tackling and blocking football. At the same time, high schools all over the country are putting greater emphasis on safer techniques and fewer full-contact practices. Along these lines, engineers are experimenting with better helmet design to protect the brain.

When played at the highest level by great athletes, football can be a thrilling and beautiful game. Some of the country's best athletes gravitate to the sport for that reason. (Bo Jackson, a bona fide all-star in both baseball and football, was quite possibly the best athlete of our generation.) If football does not want to lose its best athletes to other sports, it must make a concerted effort to temper the unnecessary violence at all levels, from youth leagues to the NFL.

The risk of head trauma in football will never be completely eliminated. Parents and young players must decide the level of acceptable risk, just as they do in other sports. But medicine, technology, sports, and common sense can converge with a common goal—to make sure football is not unsafe at any age.

VIII

CLINICAL VIGNETTES AND A
HUMOROUS INTERLUDE

63

ELENA AND ANGELA

Well, I'm not the kind to live in the past
the years run too short, and the days too fast.

—AL STEWART, "TIME PASSAGES"

RUMMAGING THROUGH MY DESK RECENTLY, I discovered a peeling old Polaroid photo taken before digital cameras were introduced, circa 1982. The picture shows a young Hispanic girl, no more than twenty, holding an infant, smiling for the camera with the old Cook County Hospital Intensive Care Unit as a backdrop. Printed in blue ballpoint on the back of the picture is "*Gracias a todos, Elena.*"

I hadn't thought of Elena in many years, but that long-forgotten picture reminded me of her story from decades ago. One morning, without warning, two residents looking for a bed for a patient suddenly wheeled the petite Elena into the intensive care unit (ICU) on a stretcher. She was in a coma, sweating profusely, barely breathing, with an extremely low blood pressure. The residents explained that she had a severe blood infection and, incidentally, was several months pregnant. Some attending consultants followed them in and confirmed that the patient had become ill very quickly on the ward; they were certain she was dying. When the nurses got her into bed, she was indeed near death.

To save patients like Elena, the ICU team—nurses, physicians, therapists—must possess two things: a firm belief that the patient can be saved and, just as important, luck. We had the former; it was too early to tell whether we had the latter.

I explained the grim situation to Elena's uncle and grandmother, as the doctors placed a breathing tube and started infusing fluids, antibiotics, and medicine to raise Elena's blood pressure. Her bedside nurse, Angela, a young African American woman not much older than Elena, was relatively new to the ICU. Angela was cheerful, always smiling, and anxious to learn, but she had never been in charge of a patient as sick as Elena. Now she approached her work with a steely resolve and a determined expression I had never seen before. If she was afraid, she didn't show it. And there was certainly ample reason to be afraid for Elena's life, which hung in the balance.

Angela was invested in Elena's care, so she took an extra shift to be with her. She made sure Elena had an experienced senior nurse to take over when her shift was finished. By the end of the day, Elena was still alive but was not much better. She might still be dead in an hour. I discussed the treatment plan with the overnight residents, but in truth there was little to do. Either Elena would respond to treatment for the infection or she would die.

I went home with trepidation, but I secretly believed that Elena would pull through. I had no choice—for patients like Elena, pessimism can be a mortal enemy.

The next morning, Elena was still alive and beginning to improve. Angela was taking care of her again. On rounds Angela knew every lab value and every trend in the vital signs better than anyone. When I asked her if Elena had improved enough for us to reduce her life support medications, Angela looked me squarely in the eye and said, "No, not yet. But by this afternoon." I thought to myself she did not have the experience to answer so confidently, but she turned out to be right.

Meanwhile luck, or providence, was on Elena's side, and she survived. Four days later, when her breathing tube was removed, the first thing she asked about was her baby. Would it survive? We told her she would be transferred to the gynecology ward, where they would know better. Then she thanked everyone in Spanish. She did not speak English, but she realized how close she had come to dying. Before being transferred, she made a point of kissing Angela's hand.

When I asked Angela how it felt, she said, "Real good. As good as any kiss I ever got." Elena went off to gynecology, and we lost track of her. We heard later she delivered a baby girl, premature but healthy. About six months after that, Elena returned to the ICU with her daughter and posed for the picture I found in my desk. Her visit was a real morale boost for the nursing staff after a particularly rough couple of weeks caring for sick patients. After that I made a point of asking former patients to visit the ICU so everyone could see them when they regained their health. That should be part of the protocol in every ICU.

Unfortunately, Angela was off that day, and she never saw Elena again. That's the nature of intensive care—intense emotional commitment and then separation forever. But Elena's case became a turning point in Angela's training.

Over thirty-five years have passed. The peeling Polaroid photo is like a never-completed jigsaw puzzle. The Cook County ICU where this happened has been gone for more than a quarter of a century now; the building, knocked down and paved over, is a parking lot today. Elena would now be nearing sixty years old, and her little girl would be over thirty, perhaps with children of her own. It's hard to imagine the smiling young woman in that picture as a grandmother. After a couple years, Angela left nursing to take care of her own children.

For a brief moment, Elena, Angela, and I all lived together intimately in a world that has vanished. Now we are separated forever, with that peeling Polaroid the last evidence that world ever existed.

64

AN UNUSUAL SIDE EFFECT OF MY MEDICINE: I CAN'T REMEMBER MY LINES

All substances are poisonous, there is none which is not a poison.

—PARACELSUS

DEAN PETER RICHARDS of London's St. Mary's Medical School was a world-renowned expert in teaching medical students to become doctors. One of his key counsels was, "All doctors must continue to learn, and not only about new advances but to appreciate the limitations of all knowledge."

Sage advice, not only for medical students but for us doddering old codger physicians as well.

I learned, or relearned, that valuable lesson recently. A neighbor suffered a sports injury that resulted in an inflamed ankle. He visited his personal doctor, an experienced physician, who prescribed a seven-day course of corticosteroid medication to suppress the inflammation. The neighbor was a stage actor, and, after three days of taking the drug, he called me from his car on his way to a local theater for that evening's performance. The reason for his call was that he suddenly realized he could not remember the precise location of the theater. He was familiar with the area and knew he was in the right neighborhood, but he was just not sure exactly where the theater was even though he had rehearsed and performed there for weeks. What was worse was that while he drove around looking for the theater, he also realized that he could not remember the lines he was supposed to deliver that night—the greatest fear of every actor.

I was afraid he might be having a stroke and I inquired about other symptoms, but he had none. His only complaint was the loss of short-term recall. As he described his problem, I was struck by how calm he sounded considering that he was due to go onstage in an hour. Eventually the GPS in his car guided him to the theater, but this did him little good since he was still unable to recite his lines. The director was forced to cancel the performance, but fortunately it was a slow weeknight for ticket sales, and refunds were not a problem.

On his way home, aided by his GPS, he called me back, wondering if he was experiencing a possible side effect of the corticosteroids. A neurologist might have been familiar with the answer to that question, but I was not, despite having prescribed corticosteroids for hundreds of patients. After consulting the Internet and my *Physicians' Desk Reference*, I ascertained that corticosteroids could indeed cause impaired short-term recall. The drug can disrupt the delicate neural connections in the hippocampus, one of the regions of the brain responsible for memory. What results is damage to what one British writer termed "the fragile mental alchemy on which we all rely."

Loss of short-term recall is not a frequently reported complication of corticosteroids, and some doctors, like me, may be unaware of it. Since so many patients take corticosteroids (prednisone is the derivative most commonly prescribed for a wide host of conditions), it follows that patients, in turn, may be unaware that short-term memory loss could happen to them after their doctors prescribe the medication.

I advised my neighbor to call his physician and in the interim to stop taking the medication, read his lines over again, and get some sleep. Many actors find that sleep reinforces memory when they are attempting to learn chunks of dialogue. Fortunately, in his case the complication was reversible, and he was back onstage and able to deliver his lines for his weekend performances.

This vignette was a lesson in many ways. All medications have side effects, and even commonly used medications have unexpected complications. Moreover, those complications have different implications depending on the patient. For an actor, loss of short-term memory is devastating. If the same thing happened to an elderly patient in a nursing home, it might have never been noticed. Even worse, it might simply have been written off to old age.

That is why it is so important to listen to what your patients tell you and make every effort to understand their particular situations. One of the other pieces of advice Dean Richards gave to medical students was that doctors "also need to learn humility, in the face of their imperfect understanding and their patients' courage." When my neighbor could not remember his lines as a result of his medication, he did not panic. Rather, he exhibited composure and poise. Exactly the type of courage the great educator was referring to.

65

TWENTY-FIRST-CENTURY MEDICINE, OR "MOM, I WANT TO BE A DOCTOR"

Man. Woman. Birth. Death. Infinity.

—Dr. Zorba (Sam Jaffe), opening from
the Ben Casey television show

SCENE: FAMILY DINNER TABLE, a middle-aged couple and their son, home from college.

Father: "So, boy, have you figured out what you want to do with your life?"

Son: "Yes, Dad, I've talked to my counselor, and I want to become a doctor."

At that moment Mother swells visibly with pride and says, "I knew it. Oh, son you'll make such a wonderful doctor. Maybe you can open up your own practice."

Son demurs politely, "No, Mom. Once I finish my training, I plan on becoming part of an accountable care organization. You understand, financial and clinical risk means it's essential to have the infrastructure to coordinate interactive team-based care. It's all about being market competitive and empowering synergistic group and management service organizations that feature mutual arrangements on optimal practice management, health information technology, group purchasing, billing/collections, human resources, and other mission-critical functions."

Mother stares at him blankly.

"Son, Dr. Kildare and Marcus Welby never talked that way."

Son stares at Mother blankly, unfamiliar with who these people are and what they have to do with medicine.

Father chimes in, offering what he hopes is a more contemporary reference, "Don't you want to be like that TV doctor, Dr. House, and make all those great diagnoses?"

"House? Are you kidding? He was a terrible physician. His style was completely dysfunctional within the parameters of a hospital environment, and he had no concept of teamwork or care coordination. Plus his show got cancelled."

Father stares at him blankly.

Mother, holding out hope, comes back, "Maybe you could be a surgeon like Ben Casey?"

Son with another blank stare at Mother.

"Who's Ben Casey?"

"He was the best surgeon on television. All night he'd be up doing a heart operation and then they would bring in some poor little boy and Ben Casey would single-handedly save him with an emergency appendectomy."

"Mom, it doesn't work like that anymore. People don't stay up all night and then operate. They have work limits now. I heard some surgeons talking on NPR, and it's a revolutionary paradigm trying to make surgical hours 'family friendly.' And this business about this cowboy Casey single-handedly saving the little boy? Don't you understand there are dozens of people interfacing in that boy's surgery? Surgeons aren't heroes anymore. Anyway, they are programming robots to do surgery. Soon robots will do appendectomies."

Mother, a little disappointed, struggles for words, "Well, I remember when that nice Dr. Green took out my gall bladder. I liked him."

A subtle eye-roll from Son.

Father chimes in again slightly irritated, "When you become a doctor, you are going to take care of patients, aren't you?"

"Dad, it's not really taking care of patients, it's interfacing with clients. Medicine is about developing mutually beneficial models that focus on shared decision-making. The idea that your doctor is the expert who knows what's best is the problem with medicine. The future is in creating guidelines and algorithms based on an evidence-based approach. The goal of medicine should be to standardize, so clients can be managed through clinical pathways facilitated by lower-cost providers."

Son grows animated, excitement in his eyes, "Don't you see, Dad? You wouldn't even need a doctor for most cases. My future could be in developing new algorithms for cases that don't conform to traditional guidelines! And I could devise new checklists. Checklists are a revolutionary approach to medicine."

Father, slightly taken aback, doesn't know what to say, so he says the first thing to come to mind, "Does that mean you won't carry a stethoscope?"

Another eye-roll from Son, this time not so subtle. "Portable ultrasound, Dad. Portable ultrasound. No more stethoscopes."

Father stares at him blankly.

Mother asks, "I just want to know if you will still be helping people and making them better."

"Sure, Mom. What you are talking about is outcomes. Don't forget I will be interfacing with the electronic health record, and it provides an industrialization function that enables us to process efficiency. Not only that, but the retrieval of clinical decisions, as well as cost and quality assessment, allows for iterative improvement. Do you have any idea what that means for outcomes?"

Mother says nothing but nods with a wan smile and offers dessert.

Son puts down his napkin and says, "Mom, Dad. I'd really love to stay and chat some more, but I have to run. I'm going to a lecture on how medicine needs to become more like the Cheesecake Factory—you know customized approach, more standardization, and enhanced quality control. That is so twenty-first century!"

Son leaves. Mother and Father finish their meals. A few moments of awkward silence until Mother asks, "Oh dear, aren't you proud of our boy?"

"I guess. But there seems to be a lot of mumbo jumbo in medicine today. I sort of wish he'd go into something with a little less double-talk attached to it."

"Like what?"

"I don't know. Maybe politics. Pass the ice cream."

66

A GUIDE TO HEALTH CARE POLICY—WITH APOLOGIES TO MORT SAHL

Liberals feel unworthy of their possessions.
Conservatives feel they deserve everything they've stolen.

—MORT SAHL

I N THE LATE 1950s and early 1960s, there was no more acute observer of the American political scene than satirist Mort Sahl. In the tradition of humorists like Mark Twain and Will Rogers, Sahl played no favorites; by skewering Republicans and Democrats with equal aplomb, he was the forerunner to today's political satirists, including Stephen Colbert and Jon Stewart.

At the height of the Vietnam War in 1967, Sahl created a satiric monologue describing the three basic political factions in the United States, the left wing, the right wing, and the moderates. In turn he further subdivided each of those three factions into three wings, left, center, and right, creating nine divisions in all, so the political spectrum looked like this:

257

Left Wing: left, center, right
Moderates: left, center, right
Right Wing: left, center, right

To illustrate his point, Sahl was able to categorize anybody's political philosophy simply by examining their stance on the Vietnam War. For example, the "left–left wing" position was that the United States should unconditionally withdraw from Vietnam (which became the official American position five years later). The "center-moderate" position was "we should stay because the Communists may strike somewhere else in the world" while the "right–right wing" position was that we should immediately start bombing not only Vietnam but Communist China as well.

Since then little has changed—the political divisions remain. Today's left wing reads the *Daily Kos* blog and the *Huffington Post*, watches MSNBC, considers Rachel Maddow their spokesman, and longs for the pre-Trump days of Barack Obama.

Sahl's right wing, now known as conservatives, reads the *National Review*, watches Fox News, reveres Rush Limbaugh as their spokesman, and anticipates the coronation of Donald Trump as king.

Moderates are currently searching for something to read, because the only middle-of-the-road publications left standing are *People* magazine and *Car and Driver*. Virtually everything else has folded or has become a house organ of either the Left or Right. Moderates have no official spokesman. They are reduced to watching reruns of *Cheers* and *Frazier* while they pine for the days of Johnny Carson and his apolitical monologues.

With apologies to Mort Sahl, here is how today's political factions, beginning with the moderates, shake out on our current hot-button issue, health care:

Moderates: The "left-moderates" favor the Affordable Care Act (ACA) health care plan. They do not believe in "death panels" and want to keep both parties as far away as possible from changing the ACA.

Moderates: The "center-moderates" favor the ACA health care plan, assuming it can be made revenue neutral. They hope President Obama knew what he was doing, while they harbor secret doubts about Bernie Sanders's economic expertise.

Moderates: The "right-moderates" oppose the ACA health care plan because they are convinced it will never be revenue neutral and will require government subsidies indefinitely. They still hope President Obama knew what he was doing, but they cast a suspicious eye at Elizabeth Warren.

Right Wing: The "left–right wing" wants no health reform. They believe our health care system is the best in the world without the ACA. Let the free market sort it all out. Everyone is on their own—as long as the stock market goes up and their taxes go down.

Right Wing: The "center–right wing" wants no health reform. In fact they are in favor of scrapping socialist government programs like Medicare and Medicaid. The money saved should be used for subsidies to the insurance and pharmaceutical industries.

Right Wing: The "right–right wing" wants to invade Canada, take over their health care system, and show them how it should be done.

Left Wing: The "right–left wing" also oppose the ACA health care plan but for a different reason. For them nothing less than single-payer health care will do. And right away by government fiat, no debate necessary.

Left Wing: The "center–left wing" also want a single-payer health care plan—and they think the military should be disbanded to pay for it. Health Care Reeducation Camps will be set up for those at town hall meetings who disagree. The first one for Camp Reeducation is Mitch McConnell.

Left Wing: The "left–left wing" also want single-payer health care financed by breaking up the military. In addition to Health Care Reeducation Camps, they want to make free medical care available to everyone in North America—Mexico and Canada included. The only people excluded from free health care, or any health care for that matter, will be Donald Trump, Mike Pence, and Rush Limbaugh. For them the only contact with the doctor will be physician-assisted . . . well, you get the picture.

Which camp do you belong to?

67

MY FIRST ENCOUNTER WITH ILSE AND ROBOT DENTISTRY

All in all, I don't think robots and greater automation
can bring about a utopian world as I imagined
it would as a kid 50 years ago.

—STANLEY DRUCKENMILLER, FINANCIER AND PHILANTHROPIST

WE MIGHT AS WELL GET USED TO IT—the future of medical care is robots. Already they are making diagnoses, performing surgery in the operating room, and soon they will be administering anesthesia. It's only a matter of time before they take over the dentist's office. Hence what my first visit with my robot dentist might look like:

It had been two years since I had been to the dentist (currently recommended interval: six months). My wife and I had to select a new dentist from our New Employee Health Care Plan. Our plan offered "complete choice concerning your point-of-care provider," which I think is medical speak for you get to pick your own dentist.

My wife was intrigued about the new robot dentist near our house. She reasoned that robots would be programmed for sensitivity and compassion. Moreover, with robots in charge, pain would be managed better, making it a thing of the past. My main concern was whether a robot would badger me about flossing. What type of artificial intelligence were we dealing with here?

Ultimately, the possibility of less pain was the tipping point, and my wife convinced me. I remained slightly suspicious that she was making me the guinea pig for this robot-dentist experiment.

I arrived promptly, and the new robot dentist greeted me with a beautiful mechanical smile. Good sign. Although maybe I should have been more concerned when I addressed it as "Doctor" and it quickly informed me, in that same unsettling voice that Amazon Alexa uses, that I should call her Ilse. First-name basis, good sign.

"All my patients call me Ilse, and you will too."

Hmmm, a little bossy, I thought, and funny that the programmers chose such an unusual name. Ilse? The only Ilse I'd ever heard of was from an old, sleazy exploitation flick, *Ilse: She-Wolf of the SS.*

The next thing I noticed, background music was coming from her body, but it wasn't traditional dentist's office Muzak; it was Prussian military marching music. Mildly unsettling.

While Ilse took questions about my dental history, another robot, a smaller fellow named Igor, entered the room, opened my mouth, and examined my teeth.

Ilse and Igor, just like R2-D2 and C-3PO in *Star Wars*. Cute.

Wrong movie. It turned out rather than *Star Wars*, Ilse and Igor were more like dentists Laurence Olivier in *Marathon Man* and Steve Martin in *Little Shop of Horrors*.

Right then Ilse began probing one of my molars and struck a deep, painful recess in a back tooth. Human dentists at least offer an apology when they hit a nerve, but none from Ilse. She just flashed some sort of enigmatic robot grin.

Then Ilse inspected my gums, my least favorite part of going to the dentist. Sure enough, she told me in a rather stentorian tone that I had not been brushing well. My gums needed work, lots of work.

Igor immediately cruised over and shined a bright light in my face, one of those lights that Jack Bauer used to shine in *24* when he wanted to drag a confession out of Russian villains. It appeared that Igor was grinning and laughing mischievously, in eager anticipation. But I know robots are not programmed for that.

When Ilse started in, my mouth started hurting—mucho. I requested more anesthetic, but she must have been designed as one of those minimal anesthesia dentists. The next hour was a blur, other than to say my best comparison would probably be what Dante must have experienced in the fifth circle of hell.

Ilse finished, and while I was still spitting blood, much blood, in her spit sink, she issued an order—nay, a demand.

"You will go out immediately and buy a new electric plaque remover."

I felt compelled to obey. Despite my pain, some strange force compelled me to click my heels, salute her, and reply, "Jawohl, Ilse, right away!"

Thus ended my first robot-dentist visit.

I left in a cold sweat and immediately bought a new $119.95 electric plaque remover. When I was a kid, it was called an electric toothbrush and cost about nine bucks. Of course back then, it didn't come with a 347-page instruction booklet. Admittedly, it was a beautiful booklet, highlighted by a full-color fold-out instruction brochure in seventeen different languages on how to brush each individual tooth.

That night at bedtime, my mouth still hurting, I began reading the section in my new booklet in Portuguese, Urdu, and Swahili on how to brush my back-left third molar. My wife came in, brushing her teeth with an old-fashioned toothbrush.

"So how did you like your new robot dentist?"

"Let's just say if the doctor told me I was terminally ill and had but a month to live, the first thing I would do is go to Ilse's office."

"Why?"

"She made an hour seem like a lifetime."

My wife looked at me curiously and said, "You know, I've decided to put off my dental appointment for a couple of months. By the way, I was reading online you should see the gastroenterologist every five years. You are overdue. I'll get the health plan and we can pick one. I think they are doing robotic colonoscopies."

"No problem, dear. But this time how about you try it out first and let me know what you think? I've had enough robotic medicine for a while."

68

THE RIP VAN WINKLE STORY AT THE HOSPITAL—WITH APOLOGIES TO WASHINGTON IRVING

Having nothing to do at home, and being arrived
at that happy age when a man can be idle with impunity,
he took his place once more on the bench, at the inn door,
and was reverenced as one of the patriarchs of the village,
and a chronicle of the old times "before the war."
It was some time before he could get into
the regular track of gossip, or could be made to comprehend
the strange events that had taken place during his torpor.

—WASHINGTON IRVING, *RIP VAN WINKLE*

IT WAS A LATE WINTER EVENING in 1970 when University Hospital's top surgeon, Dr. Elkniw, was summoned emergently to operate on a patient with a bleeding ulcer. Dr. Elkniw's specialty was ulcers, and his surgical prowess endeared him to staff and patients—he was considered a charming rogue, despite or perhaps because of rumors of an occasional drink after surgery or furtive tryst with a nurse, unbeknown to his wife.

After finishing the surgery, he stopped in the doctor's lounge to sip from his trusty hidden bottle and rest briefly before going home to his impatient wife. The clock on the wall read 1:30. The preternaturally dark lounge, and the alcohol, induced in him a deep sleep. Suddenly he was awakened by the eerie glow of a fluorescent digital clock blinking 8:00. What kind of newfangled clock is that, and where did it come from? Switching on the light, he noticed the familiar wall clock was gone.

Someone probably replaced it overnight, he thought. "Did I sleep that soundly?"

It was indeed morning when he walked the familiar hallway. Except it appeared much cleaner and brighter. Was it his imagination or were there more female doctors scurrying about than he remembered?

Straightening up in the restroom, he noticed no paper towels or soap— just some liquid gel and a blow-dryer on the wall. A dash to the cafeteria for bacon and eggs, but the woman behind the counter informed him the only offering was "heart-healthy cuisine." He wasn't sure what that was, but he was damn sure he didn't want any part of it.

He sipped a cup of coffee, which cost him several dollars. When did they start charging that much for coffee? Then he caught a snippet of conversation between two anesthesia residents.

"Go home. They can't make you stay at the hospital over fourteen hours in a row. It's a rule."

"Will do. Hey, let me ask you. Do you ever twitter in the operating room while a case is going on?"

"During long cases, I'll twitter, but most of the time I just google."

Dr. Elkniw was stunned. What are these work rules? And what type of perversions are going on in the operating room? Twittering? Googling? *I knew that some guys did some weird stuff in the OR, but that's the first time I ever heard it called that. I have to discuss this with the chief of anesthesia.*

Off to the recovery room to check on his patient. Julia, his favorite nurse, always manned the desk. Today Julia was not there. Instead he encountered an unfamiliar face.

"Can I help you?"

"Dr. Elkniw, here to see Mr. Bummel. Bleeding ulcer, last night."

"I'm sorry but there is no patient here by that name. By the way, you can't enter unless you scan your ID at the door."

Scan my ID? He had no idea what she was talking about. He was slightly nonplussed.

"Where's Julia? And who are you?"

"There's no Julia here either. I don't know any Julia. I'm Ms. Bridges. And where's your ID?"

Completely confounded, Dr. Elkniw began to doubt his own identity. Everyone in the hospital knew him. A vague uneasiness about last night's drink began gnawing at him. *Got to find my patient,* he thought.

Maybe Bummel was transferred to the ward. He hurried downstairs and searched for Bummel's chart. Nothing, no charts anywhere. He would have asked someone, but everyone was busy typing at these strange type-writers while watching small televisions. What were all these strangers doing? Who's taking care of all the patients? He didn't recognize one resident.

He corralled one of the unfamiliar residents. "Where are the medical charts?"

The resident answered incomprehensibly, "What are you talking about? Charts? We use electronic medical records."

"But, but, but . . . how do you write orders?"

"We just enter them into the computer."

Dr. Elkniw knew about computers, but they were huge machines. How could those little things be computers? He needed a pen to make notes about what was happening, but nobody at the computers had one. Not even the nurses, who always wore string pens around their necks. There was nothing to write with on the ward. And in fact, nothing to write on.

Need a familiar face, he thought. "Let me page Dr. Vedder, chief of surgery."

A resident saw him, and obliging, the resident said, "Here, use my computer to page."

"I don't know how to page by computer. Can I page him by phone?"

The resident looked puzzled, "Sure, take my cell." Dr. Elkniw took the small contraption and handed it right back to him, as if it were something contaminated.

Then the resident stunned him, "Anyway, the chief of surgery is Dr. Gardenier." The only Gardenier Dr. Elkniw knew was that dull, slack-jawed medical student who scrubbed in on last evening's surgery. *He must have some connected relative who moved into Vedder's spot. I always wanted that job,* he thought to himself.

"OK. Where's Dr. Gardenier?"

"In the auditorium. At grand rounds."

Desperately he headed to the auditorium. But it was no longer there. In its place was a new, glittering hospital entrance with Gershwin tunes coming from a self-playing piano. Someone directed him to the auditorium in a different building, a building he was sure was not there before. It was quite modern and now called the academic facility. At grand rounds, the lecturer discussed lasers and scans using slides projected on a screen without a slide projector. Like the Starship *Enterprise*. *What type of magic is this?* Dr. Elkniw whispered, "Where's the slide projector?"

"PowerPoint," someone replied obliquely. He did not pursue the matter further.

After the lecture he approached Dr. Gardenier. It was indeed the same medical student from last night. Only now he was much older, grayer, and heavier. Suddenly Dr. Elkniw noticed a wall calendar—January 2010.

"Dr. Gardenier, I'm Dr. Elkniw."

Gardenier studied him briefly and exclaimed, "Dr. Elkniw! Everyone thought you ran off with Julia years ago! Where have you been?"

He recounted his story—forty years passed in one night. His tale was greeted with skepticism, but Dr. Gardenier, with a distant memory of that long-ago operation, received him warmly. He got a hospital ID, a Facebook page, and a Twitter handle. It turned out not to be perversion after all.

There wasn't much surgery for him to do. He was now too old, and medications had generally rendered surgery for ulcers obsolete anyway. So he was granted a teaching position, having attained that happy age once described as "when a man can do nothing—with impunity." A medical patriarch, he'd entertain everyone with tales of the glory of medicine before health care reform. It wasn't such a bad life, except for the heart-healthy food.

CREDITS

Sections of this book have previously appeared in the *Chicago Tribune*: chapter 1 as "Bond Between Patients and Physicians Is in Jeopardy," December 31, 2014; chapter 2 as "Is It Smart To Skip your Annual Physical?" January 26, 2015; chapter 3 as " How Old Is Too Old," October 1, 2014; chapter 5 as "Aching for Some Undivided Medical Attention," October 18, 2013; chapter 6 as "Reporting Science Without the Drama," March 28, 2013; chapter 7 as " Dr. Oz, Heal Thyself," July 24, 2014; chapter 9 as "In Praise of First-Rate Medicine," April 25, 2013; chapter 10 as "The Ghosts of Cook County," April 11, 2016; chapter 11 as "The Man Who Saved Pitchers' Arms," March 14, 2014; chapter 12 as "The Woman Who Protected Us," November 15, 2012; chapter 14 as "Air Conditioning: A Life-Saver," June 28, 2015; chapter 15 as "Flight 191 on a Spring Day," May 24, 2015; chapter 17 as "Notorious Patients," June 13, 2013; chapter 18 as "Born to Raise Hell," May 2, 2016; chapter 19 as "Who Was Nancy Reagan's Father?" March 8, 2016; chapter 23 as "ER Overload," June 22, 2007; chapter 24 as "Protect Patients' Medical Records from Prying Eyes," April 21, 2015; chapter 29 as "The Digital Intrusion," July 12, 2017; chapter 30 as "Should You Put Your Trust in Medical Research," June 8, 2015; chapter 39 as "A Pill Not in the Best Interests," October 18, 2012; chapter 52 as "Zika," February 1, 2016; chapter 53 as "Ebola," October 29, 2014; chapter 54 as "Measles," February 11, 2015; chapter 55 as "Anti-Vaxxers," May 22, 2017; chapter 56 as "When the Avian Flu Comes," November 1, 2005; chapter 60 as "Volkswagen," October 5, 2015; and chapter 62 as "The NFL May Become Extinct," February 6, 2017.

Other sections have appeared in *Chicago Life Magazine*: chapter 4 as "The Missing Pieces of Bread Cancer," October 11, 2008; chapter 13 as "Needles to Say," February 7, 2010; chapter 38 as "Doped: Performance-Enhancing Drugs," October 11,

2009; chapter 42 as "Flying Too Close to the Sun," June 18, 2016; chapter 48 as "The New Paradigm of Assistive Technology," April 27, 2016; chapter 51 as "When the Climate Changes," April 4, 2009; chapter 57 as "The Chicago Experience with a Nineteenth-Century Epidemic," April 10, 2011; chapter 58 as "Can Science and Religion Coexist?" February 20, 2017; chapter 63 as "Elena and Angela," August 24, 2017; and chapter 64 as "An Unusual Side Effect," June 19, 2017.

Chapter 16 appeared in the *Guardian* as "Newtown PTSD," March 20, 2013.

Chapter 47 appeared in the *San Francisco Chronicle* as "How a Telltale Heart Could Change Medicine Forever," August 2, 2015.

Chapter 59 appeared in *Northwestern Magazine* as "Back to the Future," Spring 2016.

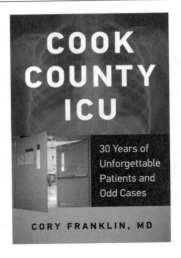

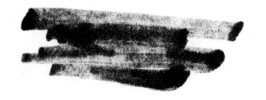

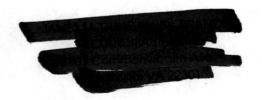